THE EVERYDAY DASH DIET COOKBOOK

ALSO BY MARLA HELLER

The DASH Diet Action Plan

The DASH Diet Weight Loss Solution

The
EVERYDAY
DASH DIET
COOKBOOK

Over 150 Fresh and Delicious Recipes
to Speed Weight Loss, Lower Blood Pressure,
and Prevent Diabetes

Marla Heller, MS, RD

With Rick Rodgers

GRAND CENTRAL
Life & Style

NEW YORK · BOSTON

All recipes were analyzed with Nutritionist Pro, version 5.0.0, from Axxya Systems.

Grand Central Life & Style
Hachette Book Group
237 Park Avenue
New York, NY 10017

www.HachetteBookGroup.com

Printed in the United States of America

RRD-C

First Edition: June 2013
10 9 8 7 6 5 4 3

Grand Central Life & Style is an imprint of Grand Central Publishing.
The Grand Central Life & Style name and logo are trademarks of
Hachette Book Group, Inc.

The Hachette Speakers Bureau provides a wide range of authors for speaking events. To find out more, go to www.HachetteSpeakersBureau.com or call (866) 376-6591.

The publisher is not responsible for websites (or their content) that are not owned by the publisher.

Library of Congress Cataloging-in-Publication Data
Heller, Marla.
The everyday DASH diet cookbook : over 150 fresh and delicious recipes to speed weight loss, lower blood pressure, and prevent diabetes / by Marla Heller, MS, RD ; with Rick Rodgers.—First edition.
pages cm
Summary: "The New York Times bestselling DASH diet series gets even better, now with this collection of over 150 mouthwatering recipes!"—Provided by publisher.
Includes bibliographical references and index.
ISBN 978-1-4555-2806-6 (hardback)
1. Reducing diets—Recipes. 2. Salt-free diet—Recipes. 3. Hypertension—Diet therapy—Recipes. 4. Diabetes—Diet therapy—Recipes. I. Title.
RM222.2.H36182 2013
613.2'85223—dc23
2012045485

Contents

Introduction

I have been cooking the DASH way (that is, according to the nutritional guidelines found in the Dietary Approaches to Stop Hypertension) every day for many years. I could be the poster girl for the diet! Not because I have written two books on the subject (*The DASH Diet Action Plan* and *The DASH Diet Weight Loss Solution*), but because I have lived the DASH lifestyle and experienced firsthand how delicious and easy the diet can be. And now *The Everyday DASH Diet Cookbook* shares my favorite recipes.

The DASH plan has positively affected the lives of hundreds of thousands of people. (For three years in a row, it was ranked #1 in Best Diets Overall by *U.S. News & World Report*, which is quite a distinction. I am also proud that the *Huffington Post* cited *The DASH Diet Action Plan* as one of the top fifty most life-changing health books.) I have talked to countless DASH fans at personal appearances, book signings, lectures, and the like, as well as in e-mails via my website. And in our conversations, recipes are a constant topic. My first two books contained just enough recipes to whet your appetite for the wonderful variety offered by DASH. I knew that cooking the DASH way was a big subject that deserved its own book. And here it is.

A few years ago at a writers' conference, I met Rick Rodgers, a prolific cookbook writer and recipe developer for many food producers. When I realized how helpful a complete cookbook would be to DASH fans, I enlisted Rick to help me put the recipes on paper. What you now see is the result of our work together—fresh, flavorful recipes for the entire family, designed for the busy home cook.

With the over 150 recipes in *The Everyday DASH Diet Cookbook*, you can put my favorite DASH recipes into action. Energize yourself for the entire day with a quick breakfast sandwich or smoothie. (You'll find some special weekend brunch treats for lingering over the Sunday paper, too.) At lunchtime, dig into a big main-course salad, topped with one of the many light salad dressings I've provided. Serve a hearty, vegetable-packed dinner with a sensible amount of meat, poultry, or seafood (or choose one of my meatless main courses). I've given you new ways to make your favorite comfort foods. Do you crave pasta? Go ahead, but serve zesty tomato sauce on a smaller amount of whole-grain pasta bulked up with lots of vegetables. You'll find a long list of simple side dishes to round out the meal, as well as DASH-friendly desserts to satisfy your sweet tooth. And to help you see how the recipes fit into your plan, I've provided a nutritional analysis for each one to help you stay on track.

Although this isn't a "fast and easy" cookbook, the recipes were created with everyday cooking in mind, made with ingredients that you are likely to have on hand or can easily find at the supermarket. The foundation of the DASH diet is plant-based foods and heart-healthy vegetable fats such as olive oil, along with low-fat and nonfat dairy, fish and seafood, lean meats, and poultry. That is a huge variety! And I make the most of it with recipes from around the world.

The Everyday DASH Diet Cookbook is loaded with dishes that you can and will make on a weeknight, without fuss but with lots of flavor. There are also "company-worthy" recipes and those to cook when you want to splurge. With this cookbook by your side in the kitchen, you will never have to worry about how to make a fabulous, good-for-you meal for the entire family.

—*Marla Heller*

Cooking the DASH Way

The Everyday DASH Diet Cookbook will become your go-to book for healthful, delicious food. The DASH diet is rich in plant-based foods, including fruits, vegetables, beans, nuts, seeds, whole grains, and heart-healthy vegetable fats. To this foundation, add low-fat and nonfat dairy (a key DASH diet food) and protein (fish and seafood, lean beef, pork, and poultry). With this huge range of options for cooking terrific meals, you will no longer have to choose between the foods you like and eating more healthfully. Based on the enormously popular DASH diet, *The Everyday DASH Diet Cookbook* is designed to make living a DASH lifestyle as simple and delicious as possible. The easier the dish is to make, the more likely you are to make it a part of your regular rotation of favorite recipes. You will, as I often do, discard the idea of a "diet," because cooking the DASH way will become a way of life, as natural as breathing…or eating!

So, what is the DASH diet? This revolutionary outlook on healthful eating was originally developed as part of a study to find ways to lower blood pressure without medication. DASH is an acronym for Dietary Approaches to Stop Hypertension, which was the name of the original study. The study organizers wanted to take the best elements of vegetarian diets, which were known to be associated with lower blood pressure, and design a plan that would be flexible enough to appeal to the vast majority of Americans, who are dedicated meat eaters. They developed what they believed was the healthiest omnivore diet plan.

And the research has borne out this hope. The DASH diet helps lower blood pressure as well as the first-line medication for hypertension. It also lowers cholesterol. When evaluated over very long periods of time, the DASH eating pattern has been shown to help lower the risk for many diseases and life-threatening medical conditions or events, including stroke, heart attack, heart failure, type 2 diabetes, kidney disease, kidney stones, and some types of cancer. Not only is DASH recommended for people who have these conditions or are at risk for them, but it is recommended for everyone in the Dietary Guidelines for Americans. And the DASH diet is fabulous for weight loss, since it is loaded with bulky, filling fruits and vegetables and has plenty of protein to provide satiety. In fact, the plan is so rich in healthy foods that people find it easy to follow without being tempted to "cheat." The DASH diet was ranked the "#1 Best Overall Diet" in 2011, 2012, and 2013 by *U.S. News & World Report.* It is widely hailed by doctors and nutritionists as the best and healthiest diet plan.

Even children get a health benefit, since studies have shown that kids who follow a DASH eating pattern are more likely to be at a healthy weight and to have healthier blood pressure. This makes DASH a wonderful plan for the whole family.

The DASH plan has its base in fresh fruits and vegetables. In this book, I use them in many ways that will make your everyday cooking look beautiful, taste wonderful, and generally be more satisfying than ever before, because you know the food is so good for you. (This does not mean that meat, poultry, and seafood are neglected.) This cookbook makes staying on track with the DASH plan as easy as can be. And by focusing on the foods to include, instead of "foods to avoid," you will develop a positive outlook on fantastic eating. Here are the tips for cooking recipes to keep you thinking positive—and looking and feeling great.

The Pantry

Have you heard the (true) advice that you should join a gym that is close to your house so its proximity negates the excuse of "It's too far to go"? You can apply the same idea to healthful cooking. If you have most of the ingredients on hand and have to shop at the market for only a few fresh items, you will find it easier to cook the DASH way. To get started, you'll want to stock some basic items in your pantry and kitchen so that you can be prepared to whip up healthy DASH recipes at any time. And I have some helpful tips that will make life easier and cooking the DASH way a breeze.

Canned, Bottled, and Dry Foods

Be a label reader! Those "Nutrition Facts" numbers on a food label can be your best buddy when shopping for pantry items. Innocent-looking foods are not always so benign. It pays to comparison shop, not just for price, but also for those numbers on the labels.

One of the most important concepts to understand is the differences among the various "reduced sodium" products. This is especially helpful for people on a sodium-restricted hypertension diet, with daily sodium intake limited to 1,500 milligrams (mg). Sometimes, a reduced-sodium or lower-sodium product might not be as healthy as you would like. A product labeled "reduced sodium" or "lower sodium" needs to have only 25 percent less sodium than the average amount found in the regular (full-sodium) version. A low-sodium product can have only 140 mg per serving. A very low-sodium food cannot have more than 35 mg per serving, and a no-sodium or no-salt product must contain just 5 mg or less.

Food products offer standardized serving sizes determined by the US Department of Agriculture (USDA) to help you compare products. For example, the standard serving size for low-sodium chicken broth is 1 cup (8 fluid ounces). A quick check of various reduced-sodium chicken broths revealed two brands with sodium contents of 679 mg and 570 mg. A low-sodium broth came in at 140 mg for an entire can (10 fluid ounces). Even with the additional 2 ounces of broth, it is easy to choose the one with the lowest sodium. With the first two brands, a cup of broth (which is not hard to consume in a meal-sized bowl of soup at lunch or dinner) would contain at least a third of your daily sodium intake! And this is with a "reduced sodium" product!

With this in mind, here are some useful items to keep in your pantry for everyday cooking:

Diced tomatoes, no salt added
Crushed tomatoes, no salt added
Tomato sauce, no salt added
Tomato paste, no salt added
Garbanzo beans, reduced-sodium
Cannellini beans, no salt added
Black beans, reduced-sodium
Lentils, dried
Canned tuna, in water, low-salt
Canned salmon, low-salt
Canned chicken, low-salt
Extra-virgin olive oil
Canola oil
Oats, old-fashioned or rolled
Chicken broth, low-sodium

The Spice Cabinet

Spices and herbs are derived from fragrant, edible plants and used as flavorings. Herbs are the leaves, and spices are the other parts of the plant, including the bark, roots, berries, flower pods, or seeds. In premodern times, spices were very expensive and rare, and then, as now, they traveled thousands of miles to get to the marketplace. These days, we literally have an entire world of seasonings to flavor our food. Make use of them! Especially in a low-salt diet, herbs and spices play an important role in the "yum factor" in cooking.

Dried herbs and spices are very convenient, and with just a shake or a sprinkle, they can add zest to your meal. Store them in airtight containers in a cool, dark, dry place. Warmth and light speed the evaporation of the essential oils in the herbs and spices, so a closed cabinet away from the stove is ideal. Even under the best conditions, opened jars of herbs and spices keep their flavor for only about six months. To keep track of the "use by" period, when you open the jar, write the date on the label.

Fresh herbs give their lively flavor to many dishes. When the weather is right, grow them outdoors, or if you have a green thumb with houseplants, try your hand at growing them in a windowsill planter. Store-bought herbs can seem pricey, but the flavor benefits are worth the price. When you have a fresh herb, plan your meals around it so it doesn't go to waste. If you end up with leftover herbs, just stick them into a bottle of red vinegar saved for the purpose to make a flavored vinegar for salads. The flavor will change constantly with the various additions, but that's the fun.

Some tender herbs, such as basil, should be stored at room temperature with their stems in a glass of water (like a bouquet); if you leave them in the refrigerator, the cold will turn their leaves black. Refrigerate sturdier herbs in their plastic containers, or if they lack containers, wrap them in moist paper towels and store them in the vegetable crisper. Before using, rinse the herbs and dry them well. Remove the leaves from the stem and chop the leaves with a large, sharp knife.

Dried basil
Dried oregano
Dried rosemary
Dried thyme
Sweet paprika (Spanish and Hungarian have the most flavor)
Ground cinnamon
Ground ginger
Granulated garlic or garlic powder
Granulated onion or onion powder
Black peppercorns
Cayenne pepper

Chili powder

Curry powder

Herb-based salt substitutes, such as lemon-pepper

Salt and Other Seasonings

The Everyday DASH Diet Cookbook is based on foods you will find in your regular grocery store, not obscure foods that you will find only at specialty stores or online sites. For those few items we recommend that may be more difficult to find, we have included a Resource Guide on page 199.

You will find that some of the recipes require a few extra spices or other flavorings than most ultrasimple recipes. In order to moderate the sodium content, we have taken a creative approach to seasoning for satisfying flavor that won't leave you missing the salt. If you have been told to severely restrict sodium, you can reduce or eliminate the added salt in most of these recipes. Because of the "flavor building" provided by the herbs and spices, you will still find the dishes to be very tasty.

You can purchase seasoning blends at the supermarket, but many of them have salt as their main ingredient. It is an easy matter to make your own at home. Just mix them up and store them in a covered container in a cool, dark place away from the heat of the stove for up to six months. They all use granulated garlic and granulated onion, which are dehydrated and ground versions of these vegetables. These have a more granular texture and stronger flavor than garlic or onion powder, but some brands of powders are actually granulated.

Cajun Seasoning

For down-home spicy flavor, use this seasoning.   MAKES ABOUT ¼ CUP

---

1 tablespoon sweet paprika, preferably Hungarian or Spanish

2 teaspoons dried thyme

2 teaspoons dried oregano

1 teaspoon freshly ground black pepper

1 teaspoon granulated garlic or garlic powder

1 teaspoon granulated onion or onion powder

¼ teaspoon cayenne pepper

Combine all of the ingredients in a small covered container.

Italian Seasoning

This all-purpose seasoning is a fine way to spice up traditional Italian dishes.

MAKES ABOUT ¼ CUP

---

1 tablespoon dried basil

1 tablespoon dried oregano

1 tablespoon dried rosemary

1 teaspoon dried thyme

½ teaspoon crushed hot red pepper

½ teaspoon granulated garlic or garlic powder

½ teaspoon granulated onion or onion powder

Combine all of the ingredients in a small covered container.

Mexican Seasoning

Here is a not-too-spicy blend that will add a Mexican flavor to your cooking.

MAKES ABOUT ¼ CUP

---

2 tablespoons chili powder

2 teaspoons dried oregano

2 teaspoons ground cumin

1 teaspoon granulated garlic or garlic powder

1 teaspoon granulated onion or onion powder

1 teaspoon freshly ground black pepper

Combine all of the ingredients in a small covered container.

The Freezer

Your freezer should be a treasure trove of ingredients for making meals. Too often it is the receptacle for bits and pieces of food that are forgotten and suffer freezer burn before they get a chance to be eaten. It might help to keep a list of what you have stored in the freezer as a reminder. Be sure to store the food in sturdy freezer bags and mark the date of freezing clearly on the package. Most frozen foods are best if consumed within three months of freezing.

Keep bags of frozen vegetables to add color and nutrients to your meals. Purchase them in bags so you can use the amount you need, and reseal either with a clamp or in a zipper bag. Avoid the ones that are laden with caloric sauces. I like the convenience of chopped onions and peppers, so I use them in my cooking when pressed for time. If you are handy with a knife, then use fresh.

Lean meat, chicken, and seafood could also be frozen so that you have a source of protein ready to turn into a meal. However, before you buy individually pre-frozen chicken breasts, check the labels: Most frozen poultry (and much fresh and frozen pork) is injected with a sodium mixture to add moisture, as the defrosted meat tends to dry out when cooked. I recently compared individually frozen chicken breasts (4 ounces each) and found sodium contents ranging from 180 to 425 mg. The solution is easy: Buy fresh chicken breasts without any additional seasonings and freeze them yourself, individually wrapped in plastic with an overwrap of aluminum foil.

Ground meat and poultry freeze well, but again, checking the labels can be helpful. Ground turkey breast, processed without any skin, is 99 percent fat-free, but it can be very dry when cooked, and I don't use it much. I would rather use standard ground turkey with 7 percent fat for moist, juicy results. (Frozen ground turkey, at an average of 15 percent fat, can have the same fat content as ground round beef, so avoid it.) Frozen shrimp, available in two-pound bags at supermarkets, are convenient and easy to defrost for a fast meal, but because they are naturally high in sodium, don't serve them more often than once every week or so.

For a treat, keep some frozen yogurt in the freezer, but be sure it's a low-sugar brand. Also, store bags of frozen fruit (such as sliced peaches or frozen berries) for tasty smoothies that can be served for breakfast or as a nutritious cold dessert.

Individual and mixed frozen vegetables, without sauces
Frozen sliced pepper and onion mix
Frozen diced onions
Frozen diced green peppers
Frozen boneless, skinless chicken breasts
Frozen 95 percent extra-lean ground sirloin (and patties)
Frozen IQF (individually quick frozen) shrimp
Frozen nonfat yogurt, with no added sugar
Frozen fruit, such as berries

Fresh Fruits and Vegetables

This is where the DASH diet really struts its stuff, letting you take advantage of the cornucopia of fresh produce available at your local market. Please—get adventuresome with your produce. I never thought that I would eat a raw kale salad (see Kale, Pear, and Bulgur Salad on page 67), but how wrong I was.

Seasoning Vegetables and Fruits

Be sure to have plenty of seasoning vegetables and fruits on hand. Onions and garlic are familiar, but shallots, a staple in French cuisine, are equally versatile and useful. Lemon juice and lime juice are fantastic flavorings and have long been used to perk up food where salt is kept at a minimum. For the best flavor, use fresh lemons and limes. To make juicing easy, use a wooden reamer or purchase an inexpensive electric juicer to keep on the kitchen counter.

Yellow onions
Garlic
Shallots
Lemons and limes

Good Keepers

These are the produce items that I always have in my kitchen, thanks to their long shelf life (at least a week, or a bit less for the romaine). Often, when I think I have nothing to cook for dinner, I am happy to find a bag of broccoli slaw in the crisper. (It can be put into service for a main course, too, as with the "Moo Shu" Chicken and Vegetable Wraps on page 112.) Baby carrots can be nibbled as a snack or cooked as a side dish. You'll find many uses for these reliable ingredients:

Baby carrots
Grape or cherry tomatoes or other high-flavor tomatoes
Romaine hearts
Coleslaw mix
Broccoli slaw

Your Personal Salad Bar

Vegetables are the centerpiece of a DASH meal. Load up your plate with vegetables, as they will fill you up and keep those hunger pangs at bay. (Although, as I often hear, people who eat the DASH plan's daily recommended amount of produce are never hungry.) These are the vegetables that I buy as needed, often for specific recipes, but also to have handy for snacking and impromptu meals:

Beets
Broccoli
Carrots (whole, sliced, or shredded)
Cauliflower
Celery
Cucumber
Kale
Lettuce (The dark varieties have the most nutrients.)
Radishes
Red and green peppers
Red onions
Red cabbage

The Fruit Stand

Remember, fruits and vegetables are the foundation of the DASH diet. Fruit in season is always going to be the best and most flavorful, but there are some items available year-round that you should always have on hand for snacks and desserts, and for adding to salads. Fruits are often overlooked as salad ingredients, but their natural sweetness can serve to balance the dressing's tartness, and they add bulk to the greens.

Bananas
Apples
Pears
Grapes
Oranges

Grapefruit

Fruit in season, such as berries, peaches, and plums

Dairy and Egg Products

Milk-based products are rich and satisfying but can also be high in fat and sodium. As you have surely seen in the supermarket, milk has fat-free (also called skim) and low-fat (1 percent fat) versions, as well as the common whole milk and (2 percent) reduced-fat varieties. Fat-free milk, which obviously has the least amount of calories and fat, is good for drinking and general use, but the slightly richer low-fat milk is better for cooking (making sauces and the like), so you may want to buy the milk that best fits your needs.

As for cheese, look for brands with reduced fat and sodium. The amounts of these nutrients will never be very low, because cheese requires some fat and sodium in the fermenting process to achieve proper flavor and texture. For snacking (or to build upon with fruit, vegetables, and nuts), nonfat yogurt and low-fat cheese are invaluable.

Eggs are another item that can be enjoyed in moderation in a balanced diet. It is the cholesterol in the egg yolk that can wreak havoc with heart health. However, most of the vitamins and minerals in eggs are in the yolks. Even the American Heart Association is now saying that most people can enjoy one whole egg per day. Many people solve the problem by using egg whites alone, but they can look unappetizing when cooked. A liquid egg substitute such as Egg Beaters can be a good alternative. If you prefer whole eggs, use eggs that are rich in omega-3 fats and lower in cholesterol.

Milk (fat-free and/or low-fat, as desired)

Unsalted butter (store in the freezer for using in small amounts)

Yogurt (nonfat)

Cottage cheese (low-fat or nonfat, and low-sodium)

Cheddar cheese, reduced-fat and reduced-sodium (Organic Valley is a good brand.)

Swiss cheese (reduced-fat)

Mozzarella (reduced-fat)

Parmesan cheese (Use in smaller amounts, since it is very high in sodium.)

Liquid egg substitute, such as Egg Beaters

Whole eggs, preferably rich in omega-3 fats

Take It Easy

Since so many DASH fans choose the plan because of problems with hypertension, I use few high-sodium foods. I've said it before: Concentrate on the foods you can have and do not worry about the few that you want to limit. There are lower-sodium versions of most of these foods, but unfortunately, supermarkets don't always carry them. (See page 199 for a list of online shopping sources.) You *can* occasionally indulge in these foods, but for the most part, limit the following:

Olives, green and black
Anchovies (oil-packed or salt-packed) and anchovy paste
Asian condiments, such as soy sauce, oyster sauce, and hoisin sauce
Prepared mustards
Pickles and relishes
Delicatessen meats

Essential Equipment

Some people enjoy cooking, and others have never learned to love it. I'll bet the ones who are happiest in the kitchen have the best pots, pans, and knives and the ones who hate cooking are frustrated by bad tools. I'm not saying that you have to go out and spend thousands of dollars on new pots and pans and expensive appliances. But a few well-chosen kitchen items will make your time in the kitchen easier and more fun. These are the things that I can't do without.

Kitchen Scales

I have put this at the top of the list because too many people consider it optional. But when it comes to maintaining a healthy lifestyle, a kitchen scale is indispensable because portion size is usually measured by weight. In the DASH diet, it is especially important to weigh your meat portions. Protein is important to help keep you feeling full, but too much will load on the calories. (There is an old trick you can use, equating the size of a 3-ounce portion of cooked meat, poultry, or seafood to the size of the palm of a woman's hand—but that may seem pretty antiquated in the digital age.) In fact, in some recipes, I have given nutritional analyses for the regular portion as well as a smaller serving for times when you are reducing calories for weight loss, or if you just have a smaller appetite.

Therefore, every kitchen should have a scale. Digital scales are the most efficient (the springs in spring-operated scales can get tired and malfunction with use), and they are surprisingly inexpensive. You can purchase one at any kitchen store or many online stores. You will find lots of uses for it beyond weighing your protein portions—for example, double-checking produce weights.

Skillets

Too often, a cook makes do with a single skillet to cook everything, big to tiny. You will find cooking much easier (and more successful) if you have a trio of skillets: small, medium, and large. Especially with meat, poultry, or seafood recipes that make more than four servings, it is important not to crowd the individual pieces when you cook. If the protein portions are placed too closely together, the steam released from the meat (or poultry or seafood) will collect in the skillet, and the food's surface won't crisp and brown. Those crusty brown bits add lots of flavor to food without adding calories.

A small skillet, measuring about 6 inches across the bottom, is perfect for individually sized omelets and for cooking small amounts of side dishes. A medium skillet, with a diameter of 8 inches or so across the bottom, will make larger egg dishes (such as frittatas) and two servings of meat, chicken, or seafood. A large skillet, about 12 inches across, will be welcome when you want to cook four portions (say, of boneless pork chops or chicken fillets) without crowding the food in the pan. And I recommend skillets with ovenproof handles, so you can use them for dishes that require extra browning in the oven.

Other Kitchen Appliances

Take advantage of the various gadgets, utensils, and tools that you have in your kitchen to get dinner on the table quickly.

Countertop grill

I often use my electric grill for quickly cooking two portions of lean meats, fish, and poultry. The newer versions have removable grill surfaces for easy cleanup.

Toaster oven

Great for making small meals or reheating certain leftovers.

Microwave oven

Always useful for reheating leftovers or cooking fresh or frozen vegetables.

Blender

This indispensable appliance purees vegetables into sauces and soups and makes great smoothies.

Food processor

Many cooks can't live without this appliance, which is useful for chopping and slicing vegetables. Just be aware that you can easily cross the line between chopped onions and onion puree, so use caution.

Mandoline or V-slicer

The mandoline is the classic hand tool used for slicing vegetables uniformly, but it is big and expensive and can be a bother to clean and store. A plastic V-slicer is reasonably priced and easier to use and store. In either case, be sure to use the hand guard, as the blades are very sharp.

Oil pump sprayer

Some recipes call for cooking oil even if you use a nonstick skillet. The problem with using a canned spray is that in addition to the calorie-rich oil, the product also contains propellants that adhere to the skillet surface! It is much better to use a pump-style oil sprayer. Also, this way you can be sure of the quality of the oil you are using in your cooking.

Instant-read digital thermometer

To get an accurate reading for roast meat or poultry, you must use a thermometer. An instant-read model gives a quick readout, and the thin probe won't leave a big hole in your food. I also use mine to ensure that reheated leftovers have reached at least 165°F, the temperature at which most harmful bacteria is destroyed.

Knives

When I teach my cooking classes, I see a variety of skill levels. Some people can chop an onion in twenty seconds, and others take two minutes or longer. People who say "I can't cook" often may just need to improve their knife skills. Get a good book (some even come with DVDs) or take a local class on the subject so you can wield your knife like a contestant on a cooking show. I speak from experience. My husband, Richard, and I took a series of cooking classes at a local culinary school a few years ago to up our game, and it worked wonders.

You need only three knives: a large chef's knife for chopping, a thin utility knife for slicing, and a small paring knife for trimming. Serrated knives are really meant to slice bread, and do not cut vegetables well at all. A good knife will last forever if you remember to hone it with a knife steel and to send it out every year or so to the neighborhood knife sharpener for a professional sharpening. There are a few name brands for knives, and all are good. I prefer thinner knives that slice easily through harder vegetables. Just be sure to pick a knife that *can* be sharpened.

Planning Ahead

We all lead busy lives these days, so look for ways to save time in the kitchen. Whenever possible, make extra food for dinner to create leftovers to serve at another meal. After all, it takes the same amount of time if you are roasting six or eight salmon fillets instead of four, and the same goes for chicken breasts. Turkey breast and beef eye of round roast yield large amounts, all the better to have extra servings in reserve. Use the following recipes to plan ahead and produce extra protein-rich foods to have on hand:

Classic Poached Chicken (page 105)
Basic Roast Chicken Breast 101 (page 103)
Roast Turkey Breast with Root Vegetables, Lemon, and Garlic Cloves (page 114)
Spiced Roast Eye of Round (page 82)
Roasted Salmon Fillets with Basil Drizzle (page 134)

Weights and Measures

Each recipe includes a nutritional analysis along with DASH diet serving groups, as opposed to diabetic exchange serving groups. Although they mostly overlap, there are some differences.

Beans, nuts, and seeds are a specific food group in the DASH diet. However, in diabetic exchanges beans are a starch, and nuts and seeds are fats.

All meat, fish, and poultry serving sizes reflect the cooked serving size, as is used in the diabetic exchanges. For example, ¼ pound (4 ounces) of ground beef provides a 3-ounce serving when cooked.

Bags of lettuce or slaw are sold by weight, not volume. For example, a 5-ounce bag of broccoli slaw actually weighs 5 ounces on the scale, rather than filling 5 fluid ounces in a measuring cup. And, certainly, you are not obligated to use bagged produce. We have provided these suggestions as time-savers, but we always applaud your use of fresh-from-the-market produce.

Any diet plan is only as good as the food that can be made following its guidelines. I am confident that these recipes will become favorites, not just because they follow the DASH diet's recommendations, but because they taste and look great.

Breakfasts

Never skip breakfast. This meal fuels you for the entire day, and it is no fun to try to make it through the morning on an empty stomach. Be sure to include protein in the meal to help keep you feeling satiated. An omelet made with liquid egg substitute (seasoned egg whites) is one of my favorite ways to start the day, since it takes very little time to whip up a hot meal. Smoothies are a popular quick breakfast, but be sure to include yogurt, nuts, or milk to up their protein content, and have them only occasionally, since they are less filling and satisfying than whole fruit and yogurt or milk. I've also included a few recipes for pancakes, waffles, and French toast for relaxed weekend brunches or when you feel like indulging.

———————

Open-Faced Breakfast Sandwich

Here's a tasty fork-and-knife version of a breakfast sandwich that you will find with many more calories at a fast-food place. You will use only half of the English muffin, so save the other half for tomorrow's breakfast or whirl it in a blender and freeze to use as bread crumbs in another recipe.

MAKES 1 SERVING

½ whole-wheat English muffin

1 slice reduced-fat (2% milk) Swiss cheese, torn into pieces to fit the muffin

Olive oil in a pump sprayer

½ cup seasoned liquid egg substitute

1½ teaspoons finely chopped scallion (green part only)

Toast the English muffin in an oven toaster or broiler. Turn off the toaster (or broiler). Top the muffin with the cheese pieces and let stand until the cheese is melted by the residual heat, about 30 seconds. Transfer to a plate.

Meanwhile, spray a small nonstick skillet with the oil and heat over medium heat. Add the egg substitute and cook until the edges are set, about 15 seconds. Using a heatproof spatula, lift the edges of the egg substitute so the uncooked liquid can flow underneath. Continue cooking, lifting the edges about every 15 seconds, until the egg mixture is set, about 1½ minutes total. Using the spatula, fold the edges of the egg mixture into the center to make a rough-shaped "patty" about 3 inches across.

Transfer the egg patty to the muffin and sprinkle with the scallion. Serve hot.

NUTRITIONAL ANALYSIS
(1 serving) 166 calories, 21 g protein, 17 g carbohydrates, 2 g fat, 2 g fiber, 8 mg cholesterol, 419 mg sodium, 370 mg potassium. Food groups: 1 whole grain, 2 ounces meat, 1 dairy.

NOTE: If you want to reduce sodium, use unseasoned egg whites; this will reduce the sodium by about 70 mg.

Swiss Cheese

I love 2% milk Swiss cheese and find it to be one of the creamier reduced-fat cheeses. For convenience, I buy packages of sliced reduced-fat (2% milk) Swiss cheese to use in sandwiches, salads (cut into strips and sprinkled on greens for added protein), and egg dishes. Even "regular" Swiss cheese has much less sodium than other varieties, but to keep your fat intake low, buy the reduced-fat version.

Variation

Bacon Breakfast Sandwich: Omit the Swiss cheese. Cook 1 slice reduced-sodium bacon according to the package directions in the skillet or in a microwave oven. Transfer to a chopping board and coarsely chop the bacon. Add to the skillet with the egg substitute.

NUTRITIONAL ANALYSIS
(1 serving) 203 calories, 20 g protein, 16 g carbohydrates, 7 g fat, 2 g fiber, 16 mg cholesterol, 506 mg sodium, 426 mg potassium. Food groups: 1 whole grain, 3 ounces meat, 1 fat.

Tartine with Cream Cheese and Strawberries

A *tartine* is an open-faced sandwich, and it is a staple of French café menus. It is becoming common at American cafés, too. Topped with healthful foods, it will keep you filled up and energized. If the berries are naturally sweet, you won't need any sweetener, but you may add a drizzle of honey if you wish.　　　　　　　　MAKES 1 SERVING

1 slice whole-grain bread

2 tablespoons spreadable fat-free cream cheese

2 large strawberries, hulled and sliced

1 teaspoon honey (optional)

Toast the bread in a toaster. Spread with the cream cheese, and top with the strawberries. Drizzle with the honey, if using.

NUTRITIONAL ANALYSIS

(1 serving) 167 calories, 9 g protein, 27 g carbohydrates, 3 g fiber, 4 mg cholesterol, 370 mg sodium, 265 mg potassium. Food groups: 1 whole grain, 1 fruit, 1 dairy.

Variation

Blueberry and Almond Butter *Tartine*: Substitute 1 tablespoon almond butter and 2 tablespoons blueberries for the cream cheese and strawberries. Press the blueberries gently into the almond butter to adhere.

NUTRITIONAL ANALYSIS

(1 serving) 147 calories, 9 g protein, 26 mg carbohydrates, 1 g fat, 3 g fiber, 4 mg cholesterol, 339 mg sodium, 142 mg potassium. Food groups: 1 whole grain, ½ fruit, 1 nut.

Bread in the DASH Diet

Did you know that bread is the number one source of sodium in the typical American diet? There is always a relatively high amount of sodium in bread, both commercial and homemade, because salt is needed to control yeast growth. (Without the salt to subdue it, the yeast would work too rapidly.)

Look carefully at bread labels to compare the sodium levels. You may like light or reduced-calorie bread, which is sliced thinner than usual and cuts sodium as well as calories. When you find a bread brand that you like, write down the name so you'll remember it the next time you shop. Store the bread in the refrigerator or freezer to extend its freshness beyond the use-by date on the wrapper.

Broccoli and Pepper Jack Omelet

Practice makes perfect with omelets. Once you've mastered the technique, you will have a hot breakfast in a couple of minutes. Leftover vegetables from last night's dinner, warmed briefly in the skillet or in a microwave before making the omelet, can be put to use in the morning to start the day. Here is a basic cheese omelet recipe with a few variations.

MAKES 1 SERVING

Olive oil in a pump sprayer

½ cup seasoned liquid egg substitute

1 slice reduced-fat (2% milk) pepper Jack cheese, torn into a few pieces

¼ cup cooked and chopped broccoli (thawed frozen broccoli is fine), warmed in a microwave

Spray a small nonstick skillet with oil and heat over medium heat. Add the egg substitute and cook until the edges are set, about 15 seconds. Using a heatproof spatula, lift the edges of the egg substitute so the uncooked liquid can flow underneath. Continue cooking, lifting the edges about every 15 seconds, until the omelet is set, about 1½ minutes total.

Remove from the heat. Scatter the cheese and broccoli over the top of the omelet. Tilt the pan slightly, and use the spatula to help the omelet fold over on itself into thirds. (The cheese will melt from the heat of the omelet.) Slide out onto a plate and serve.

NUTRITIONAL ANALYSIS
(1 serving) 145 calories, 18 g protein, 5 g carbohydrates, 4 g fat, 1 g fiber, 10 mg cholesterol, 381 mg sodium, 314 mg potassium. Food groups: 2 ounces meat, 1 dairy, ½ vegetable.

NOTE: For severely restricted-sodium diets, use unseasoned egg whites for a savings of about 70 mg sodium.

Variation

Roasted Mushroom and Swiss Cheese Omelet: Substitute ¼ cup coarsely chopped Roasted Mushrooms with Thyme and Garlic (page 172) and reduced-fat (2% milk) Swiss cheese for the broccoli and pepper Jack.

NUTRITIONAL ANALYSIS

(1 serving) 116 calories, 20 g protein, 6 g carbohydrates, 6 g fat, 0 g fiber, 7 mg cholesterol, 413 mg sodium, 536 mg potassium. Food groups: 2 ounces meat, 1 dairy, ½ vegetable.

NOTE: For restricted-sodium diets, use unseasoned egg whites for a savings of about 70 mg sodium.

Variation

Spinach and Goat Cheese Omelet: Substitute 2 tablespoons chopped spinach (thawed frozen spinach is fine) and 2 tablespoons crumbled goat cheese for the broccoli and pepper Jack.

NUTRITIONAL ANALYSIS

(1 serving) 147 calories, 18 g protein, 4 g carbohydrates, 2 g fat, 1 g fiber, 2 mg cholesterol, 318 mg sodium, 262 mg potassium. Food groups: 2 ounces meat, 1 dairy, ½ vegetable.

NOTE: For restricted-sodium diets, use unseasoned egg whites for a savings of about 70 mg sodium.

Make It Your Way Granola

There are a lot of good things about granola, but commercial versions are often fat-and-calorie bombs. It is fun and simple to make granola at home with reduced amounts of fat and sugar. This recipe includes raisins and dates as natural sources of sweetness, and you can personalize your serving by adding a tablespoon of chopped nuts or sunflower seeds, according to your eating plan for the day.   MAKES 5 CUPS, 10 SERVINGS

¼ cup packed light brown sugar

2 tablespoons water

1 tablespoon vegetable oil

1 teaspoon ground cinnamon

1 teaspoon maple flavoring or vanilla extract

4 cups old-fashioned (rolled) oats

1 cup dark raisins

½ cup chopped dates

½ cup fat-free milk, for serving

Preheat the oven to 300°F.

In a large bowl, whisk together the brown sugar, water, oil, cinnamon, and maple flavoring until the sugar is dissolved. Add the oats and mix until lightly coated. Spread evenly on a large rimmed baking sheet.

Bake, stirring occasionally and bringing the toasted edges in toward the center of the granola, until the oats are evenly crisp, about 40 minutes. Remove from the oven and stir in the raisins and dates. Let cool completely. Store in an airtight container for up to 2 weeks.

For each serving, scoop ½ cup of granola into a bowl and add milk.

NUTRITIONAL ANALYSIS

(1 serving: ½ cup granola without milk) 165 calories, 3 g protein, 35 g carbohydrates, 2.5 g fat, 3 g fiber, 0 mg cholesterol, 4 mg sodium, 250 mg potassium. Food groups: 2 whole grains, 1 fruit.

(1 serving: ½ cup granola with milk) 205 calories, 7 g protein, 41 g carbohydrates, 2.5 g fat, 3 g fiber, 5 mg cholesterol, 54 mg sodium, 440 mg potassium. Food groups: 2 whole grains, 1 fruit, ½ dairy.

Apple and Spice Oatmeal

If you like oatmeal in the morning, your allowance of 1 ounce (dry, by weight) won't look like much in your cereal bowl. With the addition of an apple to add bulk and flavor, you will have a substantial breakfast sure to keep you going until lunchtime. And believe the good stuff you've heard about oatmeal: This recipe will contribute 2 grams of soluble fiber to your daily intake, which helps to lower cholesterol.   MAKES 1 SERVING

1 sweet apple, such as Gala or Golden Delicious, peeled, cored, and cut into ½-inch dice

⅔ cup water

⅓ cup old-fashioned (rolled) oats

Pinch of ground cinnamon

Pinch of freshly grated nutmeg

A few grains of kosher salt

½ cup fat-free milk, for serving

In a small saucepan, combine the apple, water, oats, cinnamon, nutmeg, and salt. Bring to a boil over medium heat, reduce the heat to low, and cover. Simmer until the oats are tender, about 4 minutes.

To microwave: In a 1-quart microwave-safe bowl, combine the apple, water, oats, cinnamon, nutmeg, and salt. Cover tightly with plastic wrap and microwave on high power until the oats are tender, about 4 minutes. Uncover carefully, stir, and let stand for 1 minute.

Transfer the oatmeal to a bowl, pour in the milk, and serve.

NUTRITIONAL ANALYSIS
(1 serving without milk) 190 calories, 5 g protein, 39 g carbohydrates, 2.5 g fat, 5 g fiber, 0 mg cholesterol, 1 mg sodium, 243 mg potassium. Food groups: 1½ whole grains, 1 fruit.

(1 serving with milk) 230 calories, 9 g protein, 45 g carbohydrates, 2.5 g fat, 5 g fiber, 5 mg cholesterol, 51 mg sodium, 433 mg potassium. Food groups: 1½ whole grains, 1 fruit, ½ dairy.

Cinnamon-Almond French Toast with Raspberry Sauce

French toast is a delicious and time-honored way to use up stale bread. (Since French bread goes stale overnight, this technique was designed to use leftover slices from the night before.) If you plan on making French toast for breakfast and the bread is soft and fresh, let the slices stand uncovered at room temperature overnight to dry out. Remember to check the labels and pick a brand with the lowest amount of sodium. For a smaller appetite, cut the serving size in half. The fresh raspberry sauce will leave you feeling as though you've had a decadent treat, even with a more petite portion. **MAKES 4 SERVINGS**

Raspberry Sauce

2 (6-ounce) containers fresh raspberries (about 2⅔ cups), or 1 (12-ounce) bag thawed frozen raspberries

1 tablespoon amber agave nectar

2 teaspoons fresh lemon juice, as needed

French Toast

1 large egg plus 1 large egg white

½ teaspoon ground cinnamon

¾ cup low-fat (1%) milk

1 tablespoon amber agave nectar

½ teaspoon vanilla extract

¼ teaspoon almond extract

Canola oil in a pump sprayer

8 slices whole-wheat or multigrain bread

½ cup sliced natural almonds, toasted (see "Toasting Nuts," page 60), for serving

1 (6-ounce) container fresh raspberries (about 1⅓ cups), for serving (optional)

To make the sauce: Pulse the raspberries, agave, and lemon juice in a food processor or blender just until the berries are smooth. (Don't puree until the raspberry seeds are crushed, or the sauce could be bitter.) Strain through a fine-meshed wire strainer to remove the seeds. Set aside at room temperature.

To make the French toast: Preheat the oven to 200°F.

In a large, wide bowl, whisk together the egg and egg white. Whisk in the cinnamon until it is well distributed. Whisk in the milk, agave, vanilla, and almond extract.

Spray a large griddle or nonstick skillet with oil and heat over medium heat. In batches, dip a bread slice into the egg mixture to moisten, but not soak, the bread. Place on the griddle and reduce the heat to medium-low. Cook until the underside is browned, about 2 minutes. Flip the French toast with a wide spatula and cook until the other side is browned, about 2 minutes more. Transfer to a baking sheet and keep warm in the oven while cooking the remaining French toast.

For each serving, place 2 slices of French toast on a plate. Top with 3 tablespoons of the sauce and sprinkle with 2 tablespoons almonds. Add a few fresh raspberries, if desired, and serve immediately.

NUTRITIONAL ANALYSIS
(1 serving, without the added whole raspberries) 465 calories, 16 g protein, 74 g carbohydrates, 14 g fat, 16 g fiber, 49 mg cholesterol, 372 mg sodium, 684 mg potassium. Food groups: 2 whole grains, 2 fruit, ½ nuts.

NOTE: In this recipe, if you would like to cut the added sugar content, you could skip the agave nectar for both the berries and the French toast.

Agave Nectar

More and more cooks are appreciating the natural sweetness of agave nectar (also called agave syrup), collected from the agave plant in Mexico and South Africa. It is processed without cooking, making it a favorite of raw food proponents, and comes in light, amber, and dark varieties. Agave nectar has a liquid consistency that is slightly more fluid than honey and a sweeter flavor than table sugar. The most versatile agave nectar for general cooking is amber, which has a full (but not overpowering) flavor and sweetness level. Because it is sweeter than sugar, you can use slightly less.

Whole-Wheat Pancakes with Strawberry-Maple Compote

Pancakes can be a weekend indulgence with a few alterations from the original. Maple syrup is the main culprit, but it can be augmented with sliced strawberries for a healthier alternative. Do not refrigerate the compote, because you don't want cold fruit on your hot pancakes. To add more protein to the meal, top each serving with a big dollop of yogurt.

MAKES 6 SERVINGS

Compote

1 pound (1 quart) fresh strawberries, hulled and coarsely chopped

¼ cup maple syrup

Pancakes

1 cup whole-wheat pastry flour

½ cup unbleached all-purpose flour

1 tablespoon sugar

1½ teaspoons baking powder

¼ teaspoon kosher salt

1½ cups low-fat (1%) milk

1 large egg plus 2 large egg whites

2 tablespoons canola or corn oil, plus more in a pump sprayer

To make the compote: Mix the strawberries and maple syrup in a medium bowl. Let stand at room temperature to allow the strawberries to release their juices, at least 1 hour and up to 4 hours.

To make the pancakes: Preheat the oven to 200°F. In a medium bowl, combine the whole-wheat pastry flour, unbleached flour, sugar, baking powder, and salt. In another bowl, whisk together the milk, egg and egg whites, and the 2 tablespoons oil. Pour into the dry ingredients and stir until just combined.

Heat a griddle (preferably nonstick) over medium-high heat. Spray with the oil. Pour ¼ cup of the batter onto the griddle for each pancake. Cook until the top surface of each pancake is covered with bubbles, about 2 minutes. Flip the pancakes with a wide spatula and continue cooking until the undersides are golden brown, about 1 minute longer. Transfer the pancakes to a baking sheet and keep warm in the oven while making the remaining pancakes.

Serve the pancakes hot, topped with the compote.

NUTRITIONAL ANALYSIS
(1 serving: 2 pancakes with ⅙ compote) 267 calories, 8 g protein, 45 g carbohydrates, 7 g fat, 3 g fiber, 34 mg cholesterol, 264 mg sodium, 325 mg potassium. Food groups: 2 whole grains, 1 fruit.

Variation

Whole-Wheat Banana-Pecan Pancakes: Stir the batter just until moistened with some visible streaks of flour. Add 1 ripe banana cut into ¼-inch dice and ½ cup coarsely chopped pecans and stir just until combined.

NUTRITIONAL ANALYSIS
(1 serving: 2 pancakes) 278 calories, 9 g protein, 34 g carbohydrates, 13 g fat, 4 g fiber, 34 mg cholesterol, 262 mg sodium, 313 mg potassium. Food groups: 2 whole grains, ½ fruit, ½ nuts.

Cornmeal Waffles with Blueberries and Yogurt

Get out the waffle iron and make these crisp, golden-brown treats. (A nonstick waffle iron works best, as the batter tends to stick otherwise.) Substitute your favorite berry for the blueberries if you wish, but the combination of blueberries and cornmeal is hard to beat.

MAKES 8 SERVINGS

1 cup unbleached all-purpose flour

1 cup yellow cornmeal

2 tablespoons sugar

1½ teaspoons baking powder

¼ teaspoon kosher salt

1¾ cups low-fat (1%) milk

1 tablespoon unsalted butter, melted

1 tablespoon canola or corn oil, plus more in a pump sprayer

2 large egg whites

2 cups plain low-fat yogurt, at room temperature, for serving

2 (6-ounce) containers blueberries (about 2⅔ cups), at room temperature, for serving

Preheat the oven to 200°F. Preheat a nonstick waffle iron according to the manufacturer's directions.

Whisk together the flour, cornmeal, sugar, baking powder, and salt in a large bowl. In a small bowl, whisk together the milk, melted butter, and the 1 tablespoon oil. Pour into the dry ingredients and stir with a wooden spoon until just barely combined with streaks of flour; do not overmix.

In a medium bowl, whip the egg whites with an electric hand mixer on high speed just until they form stiff, but not dry, peaks. Fold the whites into the batter.

Spray the waffle iron with oil. (Do not use aerosol nonstick spray.) Pour about 1 cup of batter into the waffle iron (the exact amount will depend on the size of your waffle iron), close the iron, and cook according to the manufacturer's directions until the waffle is golden brown. Remove the waffle from the iron, transfer to a baking sheet, and keep warm in the oven while making the remaining waffles.

Divide the waffles into squares. For each serving, stack 2 waffle squares on a plate, top with ¼ cup of the yogurt and ⅓ cup of the blueberries, and serve immediately.

NUTRITIONAL ANALYSIS
(1 serving) 233 calories, 9 g protein, 38 g carbohydrates, 5 g fat, 2 g fiber, 10 mg cholesterol, 239 mg sodium, 319 mg potassium. Food groups: 1 whole grain, 1 fruit, ½ dairy.

Banana-Berry Smoothie

Breakfast in a hurry? Mix up a smoothie and be on your way…This is a basic formula to use with just about any fruit you like. If the fruit is frozen, you will get a frosty, slushy beverage; if the fruit is at room temperature, add 3 or 4 ice cubes.   MAKES 1 SERVING

½ ripe banana, preferably frozen

½ cup fresh or frozen blueberries

½ cup low-fat (1/%) milk

½ cup plain low-fat yogurt

¼ teaspoon vanilla extract

1 tablespoon amber agave nectar (optional)

Peel the banana and cut it into chunks. Puree all ingredients, including the sweetener (if using), in a blender until smooth. Pour into a tall glass and serve immediately.

NUTRITIONAL ANALYSIS

(1 serving without sweetener) 180 calories, 8 g protein, 33 g carbohydrates, 2 g fat, 3 g fiber, 8 mg cholesterol, 94 mg sodium, 578 mg potassium. Food groups: 1 dairy, 1 fruit.

Smoothies

Here are a few tips to make the best smoothies ever:

- Keep your favorite fresh fruit in the freezer. Frigid fruit will give your smoothie a slushy texture and icy temperature. A few ice cubes can be added to the smoothie mixture to lower the temperature, but don't add too many or you will dilute the flavor.

- Bananas can be frozen, unpeeled, for up to 2 months. The skin will turn black, but it is easy to peel off.

- Use a blender, and not a food processor, to make smoothies. Liquidy smoothies tend to leak through the central tube of a food processor bowl.

- To increase the protein content, add whey powder, nut butter, or sunflower seeds to the smoothie mixture.

- Sweeteners are usually optional in smoothies. When the fruit is sweet, you may not need any sweetening at all.

Chocolate–Peanut Butter Smoothie

This smoothie may taste like the most decadent shake, but it is actually an energy-packed breakfast beverage. The banana should be ripe, with brown specks on the skin, not black and squishy. If you wish, freeze whole, unpeeled bananas (no need to wrap them) for up to 2 months. The skin will turn black, but the fruit will be unaffected. Frozen bananas are easy to peel and cut into chunks.

MAKES 2 SERVINGS

1 ripe banana, frozen at least overnight

⅔ cup low-fat (1%) milk

⅔ cup plain low-fat yogurt

2 tablespoons chunky peanut butter

2 tablespoons unsweetened cocoa powder

1 tablespoon amber agave nectar (optional)

4 ice cubes

Peel the banana and cut it into chunks. In a blender, puree the banana with the milk, yogurt, peanut butter, cocoa powder, sweetener (if using), and ice cubes. Pour into two tall glasses and serve immediately.

NUTRITIONAL ANALYSIS

(1 serving) 250 calories, 13 g protein, 31 g carbohydrates, 11 g fat, 5 g fiber, 9 mg cholesterol, 173 mg sodium, 847 mg potassium. Food groups: ⅔ dairy, ½ fruit, ½ nuts.

Kale and Apple Smoothie

Green smoothies certainly look strange, but they are a way to get vegetables into your diet first thing in the morning. The kale has a surprisingly neutral taste. MAKES 1 SERVING

1 cup stemmed and loosely packed kale leaves, well washed

½ sweet apple, such as Jonathan or Gala, cored and coarsely chopped

⅓ cup apple cider

2 tablespoons sunflower seeds

6 ice cubes

8 fresh mint leaves

Puree all ingredients in a blender until smooth. Pour into a tall glass and serve immediately.

NUTRITIONAL ANALYSIS
(1 serving) 171 calories, 5 g protein, 19 g carbohydrates, 10 g fat, 5 g fiber, 0 mg cholesterol, 31 mg sodium, 460 mg potassium. Food groups: 1 vegetable, 1 fruit, 1 seeds (nuts).

Mango Lassi

This refreshing Indian beverage could just be the original smoothie. The most difficult part is peeling the mango, but I've given instructions on how to accomplish this quickly and easily.

MAKES 1 SERVING

1 ripe mango, pitted, peeled, and coarsely chopped (see sidebar)

½ cup plain nonfat yogurt

½ cup fat-free milk

3 ice cubes

Pinch of ground cardamom (optional)

In a blender, puree the mango, yogurt, milk, and ice cubes until smooth. Pour into a tall glass. Sprinkle with the cardamom, if using. Serve immediately.

NUTRITIONAL ANALYSIS

(1 serving) 235 calories, 13 g protein, 47 g carbohydrates, 1 g fat, 3 g fiber, 5 mg cholesterol, 148 mg sodium, 853 mg potassium. Food groups: 1 dairy, 2 fruits.

Mangoes

A tropical fruit that is exported to the United States from Haiti, Mexico, and other hot weather locales, the mango has an exotic aroma and luscious flavor. However, the uninitiated will find it mystifying to peel and pit. Here's how to do it:

First, be sure the mango is ripe. It should have a spicy/floral aroma and a slight "give" when squeezed gently. Place the mango on the work surface where it will balance itself. The pit, which is about ½ inch thick, will run horizontally through the center of the fruit. Use a sharp knife to cut off the top of the fruit, coming just above the top of the pit. Turn the mango over and cut off the other side of the fruit. Using a large metal serving spoon, scoop the mango flesh from each portion in one piece. The peeled mango can now be chopped or sliced as required. The pit portion can be pared with a small knife and the flesh nibbled from the pit as the cook's treat.

Papaya and Coconut Breakfast Shake

Because of its high amount of saturated fat, I tend to discourage the use of coconut, but coconut water is fat-free. (Some recipes in the book call for light coconut milk, but that is an entirely different product.) Although it is a trendy beverage, coconut water does have its benefits: It is naturally sweet, low in calories and sodium, and high in potassium. The clear liquid comes from the center of green coconuts; skip boutique brands and look for reasonably priced canned coconut water in the Latino section of your market. Substitute 1 cup frozen papaya chunks for the fresh, if you wish, a swap that also makes a slushier drink.

MAKES 2 SERVINGS

1 ripe papaya, seeded, peeled, and cut into 1-inch chunks

1 cup plain low-fat yogurt

1 cup coconut water (not coconut milk)

2 tablespoons wheat germ

½ teaspoon zero-calorie sweetener (optional)

Puree all ingredients, including the sweetener (if using), in a blender. Pour into two tall glasses and serve.

NUTRITIONAL ANALYSIS

(1 serving) 158 calories, 8 g protein, 26 g carbohydrates, 3 g fat, 2 g fiber, 7 mg cholesterol, 39 mg sodium, 703 mg potassium. Food groups: ½ dairy, 1 fruit.

At-Home Cappuccino

Don't rely on the local café to make your cappuccino when you can make one at home. An expensive espresso machine is nice to have, but you will get great results with a stovetop Italian coffeemaker (Bialetti is a common brand). These coffeemakers are reasonably priced, and every espresso lover should have one.   MAKES 2 SERVINGS

1 cup low-fat (1%) or fat-free milk

3 tablespoons ground espresso beans

Heat the milk in a small saucepan over medium heat until steaming. (Or heat in a microwave oven on high for about 1 minute.)

Meanwhile, add cold water to the bottom of the coffeepot up to the steam vent. Add the coffee beans to the basket and screw on the top. Bring to a boil over high heat and cook until the coffee has stopped sputtering through the vertical spout under the lid. Remove from the heat.

Pour the hot milk into a blender and process until foamy. Divide the coffee between two coffee cups. Spoon equal amounts of the milk from the blender to cover the coffee, then pour in the remaining milk. Serve hot.

NUTRITIONAL ANALYSIS
(1 serving) 135 calories, 10 g protein, 17 g carbohydrates, 2 g fat, 0 g fiber, 12 mg cholesterol, 112 mg sodium, 843 mg potassium. Food groups: ½ dairy.

Gingered Green Tea

If you are a tea drinker, up your game with fresh ginger added to the brew. Green tea is loaded with powerful antioxidants and is a fine way to start the day.   MAKES 1 SERVING

2 quarter-sized slices unpeeled fresh ginger

¾ cup water

1 green teabag

Put the ginger in a small saucepan and smash the slices with the handle of a wooden spoon. Add the water and bring to a boil over high heat.

Add the teabag to a mug. Pour in the hot water with the ginger. Let steep for 2 to 3 minutes. Using a spoon, remove the ginger and teabag. Drink hot.

NUTRITIONAL ANALYSIS

(1 serving) 2 calories, 0 g protein, 1 g carbohydrates, 0 g fat, 0 g fiber, 0 mg cholesterol, 5 mg sodium, 66 mg potassium. Food groups: none.

—Soups and Chowders—

Soup is nourishing and satisfying. These recipes all make large batches because it is worth the minimal effort to make a large batch and freeze leftovers to serve as a quick meal at another time. But soup often relies on salty liquid as its base, so you need to have some tricks up your sleeve to keep the salt at bay. The vegetables in the base provide lots of flavor, so you can use a combination of broth and water and still have delicious soup. Be sure to use homemade or canned low-sodium broth, or leave the salt out altogether and season each serving with just a pinch according to your taste. You can also round out your meal with fruit or an unsalted salad to fill you up without added sodium. Just skip the saltines!

———————

Old-Fashioned Chicken and Brown Rice Soup

Nothing beats homemade chicken soup, but there are a couple of tricks to making a truly satisfying pot. First, use chicken thighs, as chicken breast tends to toughen and dry out with long simmering. Also, the rice should be cooked separately. If cooked directly in the soup, it will soak up too much of the broth and make a very thick soup. (This is true if you want to substitute noodles for the rice, too.) Boiling the brown rice like pasta takes a lot of the guesswork out of the process. **MAKES 8 SERVINGS**

⅔ cup brown rice

1 tablespoon canola oil

1½ pounds boneless, skinless chicken thighs, excess fat trimmed, cut into bite-sized pieces

2 medium leeks, white and pale green parts only, chopped and well rinsed (2 cups), or 1 large yellow onion, chopped

2 medium carrots, cut into ½-inch dice

2 large celery ribs, cut into ½-inch dice

1 quart Homemade Chicken Broth (page 38) or canned low-sodium chicken broth

2 cups water

2 tablespoons finely chopped fresh parsley

1 teaspoon kosher salt

½ teaspoon freshly ground black pepper

¼ teaspoon dried thyme

1 bay leaf

Bring a medium saucepan of lightly salted water to a boil over high heat. Add the rice and reduce the heat to medium-low. Cook at a low boil until the rice is tender, about 40 minutes. Drain in a wire sieve, rinse under cold water, and set aside.

Meanwhile, heat the oil in a large pot over medium-high heat. In two batches, add the chicken and cook, stirring occasionally, until lightly browned, about 6 minutes. Transfer to a plate.

Add the leeks, carrots, and celery to the pot. Reduce the heat to medium and cover. Cook, occasionally uncovering and stirring with a wooden spoon, loosening the browned bits in the bottom of the pot with the spoon, until the vegetables soften, about 5 minutes. Return the chicken to the pot. Add the broth and water and bring to a boil over high heat, skimming off any foam that rises to the surface. Stir in the parsley, salt, pepper, thyme, and bay leaf. Return the heat to medium-low and simmer, uncovered, until the chicken is tender and opaque when pierced with the tip of a sharp knife, about 40 minutes.

Stir in the brown rice and cook until heated through, about 5 minutes. Discard the bay leaf. Ladle into bowls and serve hot.

NUTRITIONAL ANALYSIS
(1 serving: 1¼ cups) 208 calories, 20 g protein, 18 g carbohydrates, 6 g fat, 2 g fiber, 71 mg cholesterol, 540 mg sodium, 475 mg potassium. Food groups: 1 whole grain, 3 ounces meat, ½ vegetable.

Chicken and Spring Vegetable Soup

Asparagus, peas, and leeks are the vegetables that give this chicken soup a lighter profile than other versions. Finish off each serving with a dollop of sour cream—just a tablespoon will do a lot to enrich the soup. MAKES 8 SERVINGS

1 tablespoon olive oil

1½ pounds boneless, skinless chicken thighs, excess fat trimmed, cut into bite-sized pieces

1 large leek, white and pale green parts only, chopped (1 cup)

1 quart Homemade Chicken Broth (page 38) or canned low-sodium chicken broth

1 quart water

2 large red-skinned potatoes, scrubbed but unpeeled, cut into ½-inch pieces

1 teaspoon kosher salt

½ teaspoon freshly ground black pepper

1 pound asparagus, woody stems discarded, cut into 1-inch lengths

1 cup thawed frozen peas

8 tablespoons light sour cream, for serving

Heat the oil in a pot over medium-high heat. In two batches, add the chicken and cook, stirring occasionally, until lightly browned, about 6 minutes. Transfer to a plate.

Add the leek to the pot and cook, stirring occasionally, until softened, about 3 minutes. Add the broth and stir, loosening the browned bits in the bottom of the pot with a wooden spoon. Return the chicken to the pot, then stir in the water, potatoes, salt, and pepper and bring to a boil over high heat, skimming off any foam that rises to the surface.

Reduce the heat to medium-low. Simmer until the chicken is tender and opaque when pierced with the tip of a sharp knife, about 40 minutes. During the last 5 minutes, stir in the asparagus and peas.

Ladle into soup bowls, top each serving with 1 tablespoon of sour cream, and serve hot.

NUTRITIONAL ANALYSIS

(1 serving: 1¼ cups) 222 calories, 23 g protein, 17 g carbohydrates, 7 g fat, 3 g fiber, 75 mg cholesterol, 400 mg sodium, 725 mg potassium. Food groups: 3 ounces meat, 1 starchy vegetable, ½ vegetable.

Mexican Chicken Tortilla Soup

Every country has its own version of chicken soup. Here is the Mexican rendition, chunky with vegetables and chicken and topped with crunchy baked tortilla strips.

MAKES 8 SERVINGS

Baked Tortilla Strips

Olive oil in a pump sprayer

3 (6-inch) corn tortillas, cut into strips about ½ inch wide and 1 inch long

Soup

1 tablespoon olive oil

1½ pounds boneless, skinless chicken thighs, excess fat trimmed, cut into bite-sized pieces

1 medium yellow onion, chopped

1 medium red bell pepper, cored and cut into ½-inch dice

1 large zucchini, trimmed and cut into ½-inch dice

2 cloves garlic, minced

1 jalapeño, seeded and finely chopped

3 cups Homemade Chicken Broth (page 38) or canned low-sodium chicken broth

3 cups water

1 (14.5-ounce) can no-salt-added diced tomatoes with juice, undrained

1 cup fresh or thawed frozen corn kernels

2 tablespoons chopped fresh cilantro, plus more for serving

Lime wedges, for serving

To make the tortilla strips: Preheat the oven to 400°F. Spray a rimmed baking sheet with oil. Spread the tortilla strips on the baking sheet and spray with oil. Bake, stirring occasionally, until crisp and golden brown, 7 to 10 minutes. Let cool.

To make the soup: Heat the oil in a large pot over medium-high heat. In two batches, add the chicken and cook, stirring occasionally, until lightly browned, about 6 minutes. Add the onion, red pepper, zucchini, garlic, and jalapeño and reduce the heat to medium. Cook, stirring occasionally, until the onion softens, about 5 minutes.

Stir in the broth, scraping up the browned bits in the bottom of the pot with a wooden spoon. Stir in the water and tomatoes with their juice and bring to a boil over high heat. Reduce the heat to medium-low. Simmer until the chicken is opaque in the center when pierced with the tip of a sharp knife, about 35 minutes. During the last 5 minutes, stir in the corn and the 2 tablespoons cilantro.

Ladle into soup bowls and sprinkle each serving with about 1 tablespoon of tortilla chips and additional cilantro. Serve hot with the lime wedges for squeezing into the soup as desired.

NUTRITIONAL ANALYSIS

(1 serving: 1¼ cups) 194 calories, 19 g protein, 16 g carbohydrates, 10 g fat, 3 g fiber, 66 mg cholesterol, 387 mg sodium, 297 mg potassium. Food groups: 1 whole grain, 3 ounces meat, ½ vegetable.

Hearty Beef and Vegetable Soup

When you are in the mood for a rib-sticking soup but are short on time, this is the one to make. Ground sirloin gives up its beefy flavor quickly, and a host of vegetables fills your bowl. It is quite low in sodium but loaded with potassium. If you wish, add 2 cups cooked macaroni during the last 5 minutes of simmering.

MAKES 8 SERVINGS

1 tablespoon vegetable oil

1 large yellow onion, chopped (2 cups)

2 medium carrots, cut into ½-inch dice

2 large celery ribs, cut into ½-inch dice

2 medium parsnips, cut into ½-inch dice

1½ pounds ground sirloin

1 quart Homemade Beef Stock (page 39) or canned low-sodium beef broth

2 cups water

1 (14.5-ounce) can no-salt-added canned diced tomatoes in juice, undrained

2 tablespoons chopped fresh parsley

1 teaspoon kosher salt

½ teaspoon freshly ground black pepper

½ teaspoon dried thyme

1 bay leaf

2 cups cooked macaroni (optional)

Heat the oil in a large pot over medium heat. Add the onion, carrots, celery, and parsnips and cook, stirring occasionally, until the onion is softened, about 5 minutes. Push the vegetables to one side of the pot. Put the beef in the empty side of the pot and cook, occasionally stirring and breaking up the meat with the side of a spoon, until the beef loses its raw look, about 5 minutes. Mix the beef and vegetables.

Stir in the broth, water, tomatoes with their juice, parsley, salt, pepper, thyme, and bay leaf. Bring to a boil over high heat. Reduce the heat to medium-low and simmer until the vegetables are tender, about 20 minutes. Discard the bay leaf. Ladle into bowls and serve hot.

NUTRITIONAL ANALYSIS
(1 serving without macaroni: 1¼ cups) 217 calories, 22 g protein, 17 g carbohydrates, 7 g fat, 4 g fiber, 53 mg cholesterol, 395 mg sodium, 712 mg potassium. Food groups: 3 ounces meat, 3 vegetables.

(1 serving with macaroni: 1½ cups) 272 calories, 24 g protein, 28 g carbohydrates, 7 g fat, 5 g fiber, 53 mg cholesterol, 395 mg sodium, 728 mg potassium. Food groups: 1 grain, 3 ounces meat, 3 vegetables.

Lentil and Sausage Soup

Lentil and sausage soup is an Italian classic that everyone should know how to make. This is another wonderful soup that you will be glad you made as a big batch. Don't add the tomatoes until the lentils are half-done, as the acid in the tomatoes will keep the lentils from softening.

MAKES 15 SERVINGS

1 tablespoon olive oil

1 large yellow onion, chopped (2 cups)

2 medium carrots, chopped

2 medium celery ribs, chopped

4 cloves garlic, minced

1 pound sweet or hot turkey sausage, casings removed

1 pound lentils, sorted, rinsed, and drained

1 quart Homemade Chicken Broth (page 38) or canned low-sodium chicken broth

1 quart water, plus more as needed

½ teaspoon dried rosemary

1 teaspoon kosher salt

½ teaspoon crushed hot red pepper

1 (14.5-ounce) can no-salt-added diced tomatoes in juice, undrained

2 cups whole-wheat rotini or other tubular pasta

Heat the oil in a large pot over medium heat. Add the onion, carrots, celery, and garlic and cook, stirring occasionally, until softened, about 5 minutes. Add the turkey sausage and cook, stirring occasionally and breaking up the meat with the side of a wooden spoon, until the sausage loses its raw look, about 6 minutes.

Stir in the lentils, broth, water, rosemary, salt, and hot pepper and bring to a boil over high heat. Reduce the heat and simmer, stirring occasionally, until the lentils are softened, about 45 minutes. Add the tomatoes and their juice and simmer until the lentils are tender, adding more hot water as needed to barely cover the lentils, about an additional 45 minutes.

Add enough hot water to cover the lentils by ½ inch and bring to a simmer. Stir in the pasta and cook until the pasta is very tender, about 15 minutes. Ladle into soup bowls and serve hot.

NUTRITIONAL ANALYSIS
(1 serving: 1 cup) 271 calories, 19 g protein, 34 g carbohydrates, 7 g fat, 9 g fiber, 38 mg cholesterol, 618 mg sodium, 369 mg potassium. Food groups: 2 whole grains, 3 ounces meat, 1 vegetable.

Sausage Minestrone with Kale and Beans

This Italian classic gets its name from *minestra*, which means "big soup" in colloquial Italian. The best minestrone is packed with vegetables, which fits in perfectly with DASH guidelines. Black kale (*cavolo nero*, also called dinosaur kale) is the authentic green of choice, but any kale or chard will do. The beans add a lot of soluble fiber to this soup, which is great for helping to lower cholesterol. MAKES 8 SERVINGS

1 tablespoon olive oil

1¼ pounds sweet turkey sausage, casings removed

1 large yellow onion, chopped

2 medium carrots, cut into ½-inch dice

2 medium celery ribs, cut into ½-inch dice

2 medium zucchini, trimmed and cut into ½-inch dice

2 cloves garlic, minced

1 quart Homemade Chicken Broth (page 38)

2 cups water

1 (14.5-ounce) can no-salt-added diced tomatoes in juice, undrained

1 teaspoon dried oregano

½ teaspoon crushed hot red pepper

1 bay leaf

4 packed cups thinly sliced black kale (wash well and remove tough stems before slicing)

1 (15-ounce) can no-salt-added cannellini beans, drained and rinsed

Heat the oil in a large pot over medium heat. Add the turkey sausage and cook, stirring occasionally and breaking up the sausage with the side of a wooden spoon, until the sausage loses its raw look, about 6 minutes. Add the onion, carrots, celery, zucchini, and garlic and cook, stirring occasionally, until the onion softens, about 5 minutes.

Stir in the broth, water, tomatoes with their juice, oregano, hot pepper, and bay leaf and bring to a boil over high heat. Reduce the heat to medium-low and simmer for 30 minutes. Stir in the kale and beans and simmer until the vegetables are very tender, about 15 minutes more.

Discard the bay leaf. Ladle into soup bowls and serve hot.

NUTRITIONAL ANALYSIS
(1 serving: 1½ cups) 205 calories, 16 g protein, 19 g carbohydrates, 8 g fat, 5 g fiber, 21 mg cholesterol, 659 mg sodium, 703 mg potassium. Food groups: 1 ounce meat, 1 beans, 1 vegetable, 1 fat.

Canned Beans

Every health-minded cook knows that beans are good for you. They are high in protein and fiber, and low in fat, and renowned for adding texture, flavor, and variety to your cooking. But dried beans take time to soak and simmer to tenderness, and in today's busy lifestyles, cooking from scratch isn't always possible. While convenient, canned beans can be fairly high in sodium.

There is a proliferation of lower-sodium canned beans available. Look for no-salt canned beans at natural food stores and some supermarkets. Most supermarkets carry reduced-sodium beans in the most popular varieties (black, pinto, garbanzo or chickpeas, red kidney, and pink) in the Latino food section and other varieties (such as cannellini or white kidney) in the canned vegetable aisle. There are some low-salt beans in the marketplace, too.

Even if you can only find standard canned beans prepared with salt, a simple rinse under cold water removes the canning liquid and reduces the sodium by about 40 percent. I have purposely made recipes with a variety of beans to show the available options. I really don't have a preference of one over the other when rinsing does a good job of washing away almost half of the sodium. If you have access to no-salt-added beans and want to use them, by all means, do so.

Homemade Clam Chowder

Homemade clam chowder is miles ahead of overly salted and heavily thickened commercial canned soup. You can use freshly shucked clams (available in plastic containers) or thawed frozen clam meat. Clams are naturally salty, so taste your serving and add a pinch of salt only if needed.

MAKES 8 SERVINGS

1 large red-skinned potato (8 ounces), scrubbed but unpeeled, cut into ½-inch cubes

2¼ cups water, divided

1 teaspoon canola oil

2 strips reduced-sodium bacon, cut into 1-inch pieces

1 tablespoon unsalted butter

1 medium onion, chopped

1¾ cups Homemade Chicken Broth (page 38), or 1 (14.5-ounce) can low-sodium chicken broth

2 cups low-fat (1%) milk

¼ teaspoon dried thyme

¼ teaspoon freshly ground black pepper

2 tablespoons cornstarch

1 cup chopped clams with juice

Bring the potatoes and 2 cups of the water to a boil in a medium saucepan. Reduce the heat and simmer until the potatoes are barely tender, about 15 minutes.

Meanwhile, heat the oil in a large saucepan over medium heat. Add the bacon and cook, flipping the bacon occasionally, until browned, about 5 minutes. Transfer to a cutting board, let cool, and coarsely chop the bacon.

Melt the butter in the large saucepan over medium heat, add the onion, and sauté, stirring occasionally, until softened, about 3 minutes. Return the bacon to the saucepan along with the potatoes and their water, the broth, milk, thyme, and pepper. Bring to a simmer and cook over medium-low heat to blend the flavors, about 10 minutes.

In a small bowl, sprinkle the cornstarch over the remaining ¼ cup water, stir until dissolved, and whisk into the simmering soup. Add the clams and their juice and bring just to a boil. Serve hot.

NUTRITIONAL ANALYSIS
(1 serving: about 1 cup) 120 calories, 9 g protein, 12 g carbohydrates, 4 g fat, 0.7 g fiber, 19 mg cholesterol, 424 mg sodium, 308 mg potassium. Food groups: 1 starchy vegetable, 1 fat, 1 ounce lean meat, 1 dairy.

Cod and Corn Chowder

Cod is a firm fish that takes well to cooking in liquid because it retains its meaty texture. For the base, many soups use bottled clam juice, which has a high sodium content. Low-sodium chicken broth works just as well, as the fish flavors the broth anyway.

MAKES 6 SERVINGS

1 teaspoon canola oil

2 reduced-sodium bacon strips, cut into 1-inch pieces

1 small yellow onion, chopped

2 celery ribs, cut into ½-inch dice

½ large red bell pepper, cored and cut into ½-inch dice

3 tablespoons all-purpose flour

3 cups Homemade Chicken Broth (page 38) or canned low-sodium chicken broth

1½ cups low-fat (1%) milk

½ teaspoon kosher salt

⅛ teaspoon freshly ground black pepper

Pinch of dried thyme

1 pound skinless cod fillets, cut into bite-sized pieces

2 cups fresh or thawed frozen corn kernels

Chopped fresh parsley, for serving

Heat the oil in a large saucepan over medium heat. Cook the bacon, stirring occasionally, until browned, about 6 minutes. Using a slotted spoon, transfer the bacon to paper towels to drain, leaving the fat in the saucepan.

Add the onion, celery, and red pepper to the saucepan and cook over medium heat, stirring occasionally, until softened, about 5 minutes. Sprinkle in the flour and stir for 30 seconds. Stir in the broth, milk, salt, pepper, and thyme and bring to a simmer. Reduce the heat to medium-low and simmer to blend the flavors, about 15 minutes.

Add the cod, bacon, and corn and cook until the cod is opaque, about 5 minutes. Ladle into soup bowls, sprinkle with the parsley, and serve hot.

NUTRITIONAL ANALYSIS
(1 serving: 1¼ cups) 215 calories, 21 g protein, 23 g carbohydrates, 4 g fat, 3 g fiber, 40 mg cholesterol, 390 mg sodium, 775 mg potassium. Food groups: ½ whole grains, 3 ounces meat, 1 fat.

Manhattan Snapper Chowder

Manhattan Snapper Chowder has a vegetable-packed tomato base, setting it apart from the Yankee-style creamy chowder. It is important to let the potatoes cook until they are almost tender before adding the tomatoes, or the acids in the latter will inhibit the softening of the former.

MAKES 10 SERVINGS

1 tablespoon olive oil

1 medium yellow onion, chopped

2 medium carrots, cut into ½-inch dice

2 large celery ribs, cut into ½-inch dice

2 large red potatoes (about 1 pound), scrubbed but unpeeled, cut into ½-inch dice

1 quart Homemade Chicken Broth (page 38) or canned low-sodium chicken broth

2 cups water

½ teaspoon freshly ground black pepper

½ teaspoon dried basil

¼ teaspoon dried thyme

1 bay leaf

2 (14.5-ounce) cans no-salt-added diced tomatoes in juice, undrained

1 pound skinless snapper fillets, cut into bite-sized pieces

Chopped fresh parsley, for serving (optional)

Heat the oil in a large pot over medium heat. Add the onion, carrots, celery, and potatoes and cook, stirring often, until the onions are tender, about 5 minutes. Stir in the broth, water, pepper, basil, thyme, and bay leaf. Bring to a boil over high heat. Reduce the heat and simmer until the potatoes are almost tender, about 15 minutes. Stir in the tomatoes with their juice and simmer until the potatoes are tender, about 10 minutes more.

Add the snapper and cook until opaque, about 3 minutes. Discard the bay leaf. Ladle into bowls, sprinkle with parsley (if using), and serve hot.

NUTRITIONAL ANALYSIS
(1 serving: about 1¼ cups) 143 calories, 14 g protein, 17 g carbohydrates, 2 g fat, 2 g fiber, 96 mg cholesterol, 714 mg sodium, 496 mg potassium. Food groups: 1 starchy vegetable, 1½ ounces meat, ½ vegetable.

Sweet Potato, Collard, and Black-Eyed Pea Soup

Fans of southern cuisine will dig into this soup. Collards have all the health benefits of other cruciferous vegetables and are great sources of vitamins K and A. They are quite sandy, so be sure to wash them well. Many supermarkets now carry precut collards and other greens, but they still must be rinsed before using. Note: This soup is a very good source of soluble fiber, especially from the black-eyed peas. Soluble fiber helps to naturally lower cholesterol.

MAKES 8 SERVINGS

1 tablespoon canola oil

1 (7-ounce) ham steak, cut into bite-sized pieces

1 large yellow onion, chopped

2 cloves garlic, minced

1 quart Homemade Chicken Broth (page 38)

3 cups water

1 pound sweet potatoes (yams), peeled and cut into ½-inch dice

½ teaspoon salt

½ teaspoon crushed hot red pepper

4 packed cups thinly sliced collard greens (wash well and remove thick stems before slicing)

1 cup frozen black-eyed peas

Heat the oil in a large pot over medium heat. Add the ham and cook, stirring occasionally, until lightly browned, about 3 minutes. Add the onion and garlic and cook, stirring, until the onion softens, about 5 minutes.

Add the broth, water, sweet potatoes, salt, and hot pepper and bring to a boil over high heat. Return the heat to medium and cook at a low boil until the sweet potatoes begin to soften, about 10 minutes. Stir in the collards and black-eyed peas and cook until the greens and sweet potatoes are tender, about 10 minutes longer. Ladle into soup bowls and serve hot.

NUTRITIONAL ANALYSIS
(1 serving: 1¼ cups) 172 calories, 11 g protein, 24 g carbohydrates, 4 g fat, 4 g fiber, 11 mg cholesterol, 547 mg sodium, 440 mg potassium. Food groups: 1 ounce meat, 1½ starchy vegetables.

Homemade Chicken Broth

Chefs rarely add salt to broth because they use it as an ingredient, and the finished dish will be seasoned with salt before serving. Even though there are good commercial broths (or stocks, which are essentially the same thing) for sale, making your own is easy and worthwhile. Refrigerate the stock overnight so the fat can be removed from the surface. Then divide the broth into convenient 1-cup, 2-cup, or 4-cup freezer-safe containers and freeze your batch for months.

MAKES ABOUT 3 QUARTS

3½ pounds chicken wings or backs

1 tablespoon vegetable oil

1 medium yellow onion, chopped

1 medium carrot, chopped

1 medium celery rib, chopped

About 4½ quarts water, divided

4 fresh parsley sprigs

½ teaspoon black peppercorns

¼ teaspoon dried thyme

1 bay leaf

Preheat the oven to 450°F.

Using a cleaver or a heavy knife, chop the wings into pieces between the joints. (Chopping the backs into 2- or 3-inch chunks is optional.) Spread in a large roasting pan. Roast until the wings are nicely browned, about 40 minutes.

Meanwhile, heat the oil in a large stockpot over medium heat. Add the onion, carrot, and celery and cook, stirring occasionally, until softened, about 5 minutes. Using tongs, transfer the wings to the pot.

Pour out any fat in the roasting pan. Place the pan over two burners on high heat and heat until the pan is sizzling. Add 2 cups of the water and bring to a boil, scraping up the browned bits in the pan with a wooden spoon. Pour into the pot and add enough cold water (about 4 quarts) to cover the ingredients by 1 inch. Increase the heat under the pot and bring just to a boil, using a large spoon to skim off any foam that rises to the surface.

Reduce the heat to low. Add the parsley, peppercorns, thyme, and bay leaf. Simmer, uncovered, until the stock is well flavored, at least 2 hours and up to 4 hours.

Place a colander in a very large heatproof bowl. Strain the broth into the bowl, discarding the solids in the colander. Position the bowl of broth into a larger bowl of ice water. Let the broth stand, stirring occasionally, until tepid, about 30 minutes. Remove the bowl from the ice water, place on a kitchen towel, and dry the sides of the bowl. Refrigerate, uncovered, overnight.

Using a spoon, scrape off the fat from the surface of the broth. (The broth can be refrigerated for up to 3 days or transferred to airtight containers and frozen for up to 3 months.)

NUTRITIONAL ANALYSIS
(1 cup) 10 calories, 2 g protein, 0 g carbohydrates, 0 g fat, 0 g fiber, 0 mg cholesterol, 60 mg sodium, 204 mg potassium. Food groups: none.

Variation

Homemade Beef Stock: Substitute 3 pounds of beef soup bones and 1 pound beef shin for the chicken wings.

NUTRITIONAL ANALYSIS
(1 cup) 38 calories, 5 g protein, 0 g carbohydrates, 1 g fat, 0 g fiber, 0 mg cholesterol, 25 mg sodium, 206 mg potassium. Food groups: 1 ounce meat.

Sodium in Canned Broth

Looking for low-sodium broth can be quite an education in label reading. Remember that there is a difference between reduced-sodium, lower-sodium, and low-sodium products. If you are looking for a true low-sodium broth, be sure that it is clearly stated as such on the packaging and that the nutritional label shows less than 150 mg sodium per cup of broth. Even no-sodium broths will have some naturally occurring sodium. If you use them, you can adjust the salt in your cooking as needed.

Big and Small Salads

Fruits and vegetables are key to most of the many health benefits of the DASH diet: They are bulky and filling, while mostly being relatively low in calories for their size. The salads in this chapter are appetizingly fresh and colorful, and you know that this is the plan for you just looking at them. For too long, many Americans considered salads to be a minor component in a meal heavy with meat and starch. The tide has turned, and more people are serving and savoring main-course salads. This chapter has everything from crowd-pleasers like *salade Niçoise* and Chinese Chicken Salad to more unusual offerings with fruit and seafood. In most cases, I've added a protein to be sure that you will feel satiated after your meal. Many of the meat-based salads (chicken, turkey, and tuna) can be used for open-faced sandwiches, too. You'll also find lighter, meatless salads to help round out meals and a range of reduced-fat salad dressings (see pages 72 to 74) from thick and creamy varieties to tart vinaigrettes.

Roast Beef Salad with Beets, Apple, and Horseradish

Based on a Scandinavian recipe, this salad is sweet, tart, crunchy, and meaty all at once. Once you become accustomed to fresh horseradish, you may not go back to the bottled variety. Peeled and shredded horseradish gets hotter as it stands exposed to the air, so for the mildest flavor, use right after preparation. Leftover horseradish can be grated and covered with cider vinegar to make a homemade condiment that will keep, refrigerated, for months.   MAKES 4 SERVINGS

4 medium beets (1 pound), scrubbed but unpeeled

2 tablespoons cider vinegar

1½ tablespoons pared and freshly grated horseradish (use a zester, such as a Microplane)

2 tablespoons olive oil

1 large Rome apple, cored and cut into ½-inch dice

1 scallion, white and green parts, finely chopped

12 ounces thinly sliced Spiced Roast Eye of Round (page 82)

Preheat the oven to 400°F. Wrap each beet in aluminum foil and place on a rimmed baking sheet. Bake until the beets are tender when pierced with the tip of a small, sharp knife, about 1¼ hours. Unwrap and let cool. Peel the beets and cut into ½-inch dice.

In a medium bowl, whisk together the vinegar and horseradish, then whisk in the oil. Add the beets, apple, and scallion and mix well. Cover and refrigerate until chilled, at least 1 hour or up to 1 day.

Divide the beet salad among four dinner plates and top with equal amounts of the sliced roast beef. Serve chilled.

NUTRITIONAL ANALYSIS
(1 serving) 285 calories, 27 g protein, 21 g carbohydrates, 11 g fat, 5 g fiber, 62 mg cholesterol, 185 mg sodium, 675 mg potassium. Food groups: 3 ounces meat, ½ fruit, 1 starchy vegetable.

Transporting Salads

If you want to bring your salad to work, avoid the soggy salad syndrome. Outfit yourself with an insulated lunch box with a cold pack (check out www.lunchboxes.com for a great selection) and a collection of covered plastic containers or zippered plastic bags. Pack the greens, meat, and dressing separately, and combine them just before serving.

Classic Chicken Salad with Romaine

In a sandwich or salad, this chunky mixture of chicken and vegetables is hard to surpass for old-fashioned goodness. See the variations for spicier alternatives. MAKES 2 SERVINGS

2 tablespoons light mayonnaise

2 tablespoons plain low-fat yogurt

¼ teaspoon kosher salt (optional)

⅛ teaspoon freshly ground black pepper

8 ounces Basic Roast Chicken Breast 101 or Classic Poached Chicken (page 103 or 105), cut into ½-inch dice (1½ cups)

2 small celery ribs, finely diced

1 scallion, white and green parts, finely chopped

4 romaine lettuce leaves, for serving

In a medium bowl, combine the mayonnaise, yogurt, salt (if using), and pepper. Add the chicken, celery, and scallion and mix well. (The salad can be refrigerated in a covered container for up to 2 days.)

Spoon equal portions of the chicken salad onto two plates, add the lettuce, and serve.

NUTRITIONAL ANALYSIS
(1 serving) 197 calories, 25 g protein, 4 g carbohydrates, 8 g fat, 1 g fiber, 79 mg cholesterol, 276 mg sodium, 588 mg potassium. Food groups: 4 ounces meat.

NOTE: Total with optional salt is 522 mg sodium per serving.

Variation

Indian Curried Chicken Salad: Substitute 1 Granny Smith apple, peeled, cored, and finely diced, for the celery. Add 1 teaspoon curry powder.

NUTRITIONAL ANALYSIS
(1 serving) 221 calories, 25 g protein, 11 g carbohydrates, 8 g fat, 1 g fiber, 79 mg cholesterol, 244 mg sodium, 541 mg potassium. Food groups: 4 ounces meat, ½ fruit.

NOTE: Total with optional salt is 490 mg sodium per serving.

Variation

Thai Curried Chicken Salad: Omit the pepper and the salt. Add 1 teaspoon Thai red curry paste (or more to taste) to the mayonnaise mixture. Stir in ⅓ cup coarsely chopped roasted and unsalted cashews.

NUTRITIONAL ANALYSIS
(1 serving) 333 calories, 28 mg protein, 12 g carbohydrates, 19 g fat, 2 g fiber, 79 mg cholesterol, 226 mg sodium, 708 mg potassium. Food groups: 4 ounces meat, 1 nuts.

Some Fat, Not No Fat

Remember that you need a moderate amount of fat in your diet for health and to make the meals more satisfying, tasty, and filling. Salad dressings using olive and canola oil are a good way to include heart-healthy fats in your meals. That doesn't give you a free ticket to eat unlimited amounts of fat. If your salad is dressed, you may need to balance the meal with other components that are lower in fat, such as fish or skinless poultry.

Chinese Chicken Salad

Asian flavors abound in this filling, multihued salad. Cilantro haters (you know who you are) can substitute mint. If you wish, top each serving with 1 tablespoon chopped dry-roasted peanuts for an additional 53 calories, 2 g protein, 5 g fat, 1 mg sodium, and 60 mg potassium.

MAKES 2 SERVINGS

2 cups packed, shredded Napa cabbage

8 ounces Basic Roast Chicken Breast 101 or Classic Poached Chicken (page 103 or 105), cut into ½-inch dice (1½ cups)

1 large carrot, shredded on the large holes of a box grater

½ medium red bell pepper, cored and cut into thin strips

2 tablespoons finely chopped fresh cilantro, plus more for sprinkling

Asian Ginger Dressing (page 72)

In a medium bowl, mix well the Napa cabbage, chicken, carrot, bell pepper, and 2 tablespoons cilantro. Stir in the dressing. Divide the salad between two bowls, sprinkle with additional cilantro, and serve chilled.

NUTRITIONAL ANALYSIS
(1 serving) 335 calories, 26 g protein, 14 g carbohydrates, 20 g fat, 4 g fiber, 68 mg cholesterol, 760 mg sodium, 966 mg potassium. Food groups: 4 ounces meat, 2 vegetables, 3 fats.

Tarragon Chicken Salad with Grapes and Almonds

This salad is a variation on the Waldorf salad theme, with juicy grapes standing in for the traditional apples. It is worth planting tarragon in a window box or garden to have it on hand for recipes like this one, as dried tarragon isn't half as good as fresh.

MAKES 2 SERVINGS

3 tablespoons plain low-fat yogurt

2 tablespoons light mayonnaise

2 teaspoons finely chopped fresh tarragon

Pinch of kosher salt

¼ teaspoon freshly ground black pepper

8 ounces Basic Roast Chicken Breast 101 or Classic Poached Chicken (page 103 or 105), cut into ½-inch dice (1½ cups)

1 cup halved red or green seedless grapes

2 medium celery ribs, thinly sliced

¼ cup sliced almonds, toasted (see "Toasting Nuts," page 60)

2 cups (2 ounces) mixed salad greens

Lemon wedges, for serving

In a medium bowl, whisk the yogurt, mayonnaise, tarragon, salt, and pepper. Add the chicken, grapes, celery, and almonds and mix well.

Divide the salad greens between two salad bowls. Top each with half of the chicken mixture. Serve immediately with the lemon wedges for squeezing the juice over the salad.

NUTRITIONAL ANALYSIS
(1 serving) 352 calories, 29 g protein, 22 g carbohydrates, 17 g fat, 3 g fiber, 74 mg cholesterol, 658 mg sodium, 877 mg potassium. Food groups: 4 ounces meat, 1 vegetable, ½ fruit, ½ nuts, 2 fats.

Chipotle Chicken Chili Taco Salad

The smoky flavor of chipotle adds character to this versatile chili. It is much more than a salad topping: It can become a filling for soft tacos (roll it up into warm flour or corn tortillas) or be served on its own over brown rice or macaroni as a "bowl of red." You can embellish this with a tablespoon or two of salsa, if you wish. For a spicier chili, add 1 teaspoon of the canned adobo sauce from the chipotle.   MAKES 6 SERVINGS

Baked Tortilla Chips

Olive oil in a pump sprayer

3 (6-inch) corn tortillas, cut into eighths to make 24 wedges

Salad

1 tablespoon olive oil

1 pound boneless, skinless chicken thighs, trimmed, cut into 1-inch pieces

1 medium yellow onion, chopped

1 large red bell pepper, cored and cut into ½-inch dice

2 cloves garlic, minced

1 teaspoon dried oregano

1 teaspoon ground cumin

¼ teaspoon kosher salt

1 (14.5-ounce) can no-salt-added diced tomatoes, drained

⅓ cup water

1 canned chipotle chili in adobo, minced

1 (15-ounce) can 50 percent reduced-sodium black beans, drained and rinsed

To make the tortilla chips: Preheat the oven to 400°F. Spray a rimmed baking sheet with oil. Spread the tortilla strips on the baking sheet and spray with oil. Bake, stirring occasionally, until crisp and golden brown, about 10 minutes. Let cool.

To make the salad: Heat 1 teaspoon of the oil in a large nonstick skillet over medium-high heat. Add the chicken and cook, stirring occasionally, until lightly browned, about 5 minutes. Transfer to a plate.

Heat the remaining 2 teaspoons oil in the skillet. Sauté the onion, bell pepper, and garlic, stirring occasionally, until tender, about 5 minutes. Stir in the oregano, cumin, and salt. Add the tomatoes, water, and chipotle and bring to a simmer. Return the chicken to the skillet. Reduce the heat to low, cover the skillet, and simmer until the chicken is tender and opaque throughout, about 35 minutes. During the last 5 minutes, stir in the black beans. Let cool for 10 minutes.

Divide the lettuce among six serving bowls and top with chili. Add 4 tortilla chips to each bowl, top with 1 tablespoon of the sour cream, and sprinkle with cilantro. Serve warm with the lime wedges.

1 head iceberg lettuce, cored and torn
into bite-sized pieces

6 tablespoons low-fat sour cream, for
serving

½ cup chopped fresh cilantro, for
serving

Lime wedges, for serving

NUTRITIONAL ANALYSIS

(1 serving) 263 calories, 20 g protein, 32 g carbohy-drates, 10 g fat, 8 g fiber, 63 mg cholesterol, 484 mg sodium, 446 mg potassium. Food groups: 2½ ounces meat, ½ beans, ½ whole grain, 1 vegetable.

Chipotles

Canned chipotle chilies are smoked jalapeños packed in a spicy chili sauce called adobo. Leftover chipotles and sauce can be transferred from the can to a small airtight container and refrigerated for up to 2 months. Or, to freeze them, place each chipotle on a waxed paper–lined baking sheet and spoon some of the adobo over each chili. Freeze until solid. Remove each chili with its sauce from the baking sheet and store in a zippered plastic bag for up to 3 months.

Cobb Salad

The Brown Derby in Hollywood made the Cobb salad famous. Invented by the restaurant's owner, it has deceived many diners who order it thinking it is light fare. Even though this is a high-fat meal, it has 19 grams of heart-healthy monounsaturated fats. You could cut the fat content (and calories) by eliminating the blue cheese.   MAKES 2 SERVINGS

5 cups (4 ounces) mixed salad greens

8 ounces cooked chicken breast, such as Basic Roast Chicken Breast 101 (page 103), thinly sliced across the grain

1 ripe avocado, pitted, peeled, and sliced

1 cup Roasted Mushrooms with Thyme and Garlic (page 172)

12 grape tomatoes

6 tablespoons Mustard Vinaigrette (page 73)

2 tablespoons crumbled reduced-fat blue cheese

Divide the salad greens between two deep salad bowls. Top each with half of the chicken, avocado, mushrooms, and tomatoes, arranging each ingredient in its own section of the bowl.

Drizzle each salad with 3 tablespoons Mustard Vinaigrette and sprinkle with 1 tablespoon of blue cheese. Serve immediately.

NUTRITIONAL ANALYSIS

(1 serving) 438 calories, 23 g protein, 19 g carbohydrates, 33 g fat, 8 g fiber, 45 mg cholesterol, 994 mg sodium, 1,534 mg potassium. Food groups: 3 vegetables, 3 ounces meat, 1 dairy, 3 fats.

Autumn Turkey Salad with Apples and Dried Cranberries

Leftover holiday turkey can be turned into this variation on the Waldorf salad theme, which is almost endlessly versatile. Use any seeds or nuts you fancy (pumpkin seeds or pecans would also be great) or raisins or dried sweet cherries instead of dried cranberries. Don't bother to peel the apples; the skin is good for you and adds color to the salad. This makes a very good sandwich filling, too.   MAKES 4 SERVINGS

¼ cup buttermilk

2 tablespoons light mayonnaise

¼ teaspoon kosher salt

¼ teaspoon freshly ground black pepper

10 ounces cooked turkey breast, such as Roast Turkey Breast with Root Vegetables, Lemon, and Garlic Cloves (page 114), cut into ½-inch dice (2 cups)

2 sweet apples, such as Gala or Fuji, cored and cut into ½-inch dice

¼ cup dried cranberries

¼ cup unsalted raw sunflower seeds

5 cups (4 ounces) mixed salad greens

In a medium bowl, whisk together the buttermilk, mayonnaise, salt, and pepper. Add the turkey, apples, dried cranberries, and sunflower seeds and mix well. (The salad may be stored refrigerated in a covered container for up to 1 day.)

Divide the greens among four salad bowls. Top each with equal amounts of the salad and serve immediately.

NUTRITIONAL ANALYSIS

(1 serving) 233 calories, 20 g protein, 22 g carbohydrates, 8 g fat, 4 g fiber, 47 mg cholesterol, 215 mg sodium, 440 mg potassium. Food groups: 3 ounces meat, 1 vegetable, 1½ fruits, ½ nuts.

Salmon *Salade Niçoise*

Salade Niçoise is a terrific main-course salad, but it can be improved by replacing the usual canned tuna with fresh salmon. (Of course, in a pinch you could use 2 drained cans of low-sodium tuna.)   MAKES 4 SERVINGS

6 ounces green beans, trimmed and cut into 1-inch lengths (see note)

2 medium Yukon Gold potatoes (8 ounces), scrubbed, unpeeled, and cut into ½-inch-thick rounds

1 recipe Lemon Vinaigrette (page 73), divided

2 scallions, white parts finely chopped and green parts sliced

6 cups (5 ounces) mixed salad greens, such as mesclun

1 cup halved grape tomatoes

4 roasted salmon fillets (see Roasted Salmon Fillets with Basil Drizzle, page 134, for instructions)

Bring a medium saucepan of water to a boil over high heat. Add the green beans and cook until crisp-tender, about 3 minutes. Lift them out of the water with a wire sieve or slotted spoon and transfer to a colander. Rinse under cold running water and set aside.

Add the potatoes to the water and reduce the heat to medium. Cook until the potatoes are just tender, about 15 minutes. Drain and rinse under cold running water. Transfer to a bowl. Add 1 tablespoon of the vinaigrette and the chopped scallion whites and mix. Let the potato salad cool to room temperature.

In a large bowl, toss the salad greens, tomatoes, and green beans with the remaining vinaigrette. Spread on a platter and top with the roasted salmon fillets. Arrange the potato salad in four portions on the platter. Sprinkle with the scallion greens and serve.

NUTRITIONAL ANALYSIS

(1 serving) 393 calories, 37 g protein, 19 g carbohydrates, 18 g fat, 5 g fiber, 94 mg cholesterol, 494 mg sodium, 1,415 mg potassium. Food groups: 5 ounces meat, ½ starchy vegetable, 3 vegetables, 1 fat.

NOTE: If you wish to be more authentically French, use the thin green beans known as haricots verts. Because the quality of fresh beans is iffy outside of my local summer growing season, I often prefer to buy frozen haricots verts from my local warehouse club store or the C&W brand, which may be found at many supermarkets.

Warm Spinach Salad with Scallops and Oranges

Sweet scallops, seared to caramelize their surfaces, are tossed with verdant green baby spinach and bright orange segments to make an appealing main-course salad.

MAKES 4 SERVINGS

Vinaigrette

2 large navel oranges

2 tablespoons olive oil

2 tablespoons minced shallots

1 tablespoon balsamic vinegar

¼ teaspoon kosher salt

¼ teaspoon freshly ground black pepper

Salad

⅓ cup raw unsalted sunflower seeds

Olive oil in a spray pump

1 pound sea scallops, cut in half crosswise

7½ cups (6 ounces) baby spinach

To make the vinaigrette: Grate the zest from 1 orange into a small bowl. Using a serrated knife, trim the top and bottom off the other orange so it stands on the work counter. Cut off the thick peel where it meets the flesh so you end up with a skinless sphere. Then, working over a medium bowl to catch the juices, hold the fruit in one hand and cut between the thin membranes to release the segments, letting them fall into the bowl. Repeat with the remaining orange. Squeeze the juices from the membranes into the bowl. Measure and reserve 2 tablespoons of orange juice, then set aside the orange juice and orange segments.

Heat the oil in a large nonstick skillet over medium heat. Add the shallots and sauté until softened, about 1 minute. Remove from the heat. Stir in the vinegar and orange juice. Using a heatproof spatula, scrape the mixture into the bowl with the orange zest. Add the salt and pepper and whisk well.

To make the salad: Wipe the skillet clean with paper towels. Heat the skillet over medium heat. Add the sunflower seeds and cook, stirring often, until fragrant and toasted, about 2 minutes. Turn out onto a plate.

Spray the skillet with oil and heat over medium-high heat. Add the scallops and cook, turning halfway through cooking, until seared on both sides, about 3 minutes.

Combine the spinach and orange segments in a large bowl. Add the scallops, vinaigrette, and sunflower seeds and toss. Serve warm.

NUTRITIONAL ANALYSIS

(1 serving) 271 calories, 18 g protein, 21 g carbohydrates, 14 g fat, 4 g fiber, 27 mg cholesterol, 736 mg sodium, 748 mg potassium. Food groups: 2½ ounces meat, 1½ vegetables, 2 fruits, ½ nuts, 1 fat.

NOTE: If you are watching sodium, cut the salt to ¼ teaspoon for a total of 603 mg sodium per serving; eliminating the salt reduces it to 480 mg. Most of the salt comes from the scallops, which come from salty ocean water.

Shrimp, Mango, and Black Bean Salad

The striking good looks of this salad are a preview to its rich flavor. You could use steamed shrimp, but grilled (or broiled) shrimp somehow pair best with the mango and black beans. You should note that the actual sodium in the dish will be lower than shown here, because you will rinse and drain the beans, which will reduce the sodium by about 100 mg per serving.   MAKES 4 SERVINGS

2 tablespoons olive oil, plus more in a pump sprayer

¾ pound large shrimp (16 to 20), peeled and deveined

2 tablespoons fresh lime juice

2 ripe mangoes, pitted, peeled, and cut into ½-inch dice (see page 18)

1 (15-ounce) can reduced-sodium black beans, drained and rinsed

½ jalapeño, seeded and minced

2 tablespoons finely chopped fresh cilantro or mint

2 tablespoons minced red onion

Spray a large ridged grill pan with oil and heat over medium heat. Add the shrimp to the pan. (Or position a broiler rack about 4 inches from the source of heat and preheat the broiler. Spray the broiler rack with oil and spread the shrimp on the rack.) Cook, turning occasionally, until the shrimp are opaque throughout, 3 to 5 minutes. Refrigerate to cool completely, about 20 minutes.

In a large serving bowl, whisk together the lime juice and the 2 tablespoons oil. Add the shrimp, mango, beans, jalapeño, cilantro, and onion and toss gently. Serve immediately.

NUTRITIONAL ANALYSIS

(1 serving) 213 calories, 18 g protein, 36 g carbohydrates, 2 g fat, 7 g fiber, 107 mg cholesterol, 679 mg sodium, 686 mg potassium. Food groups: 2½ ounces meat, 1 beans, 1 fruit, 1 fat.

Watermelon, Basil, and Shrimp Salad

Watermelon's firm texture and refreshing flavor make it a natural for salads. This sophisticated and intriguing combination of ingredients is just the thing for a summer meal. It is best when served ice cold. As with most shrimp dishes, the majority of the sodium comes from the shrimp, so enjoy this as a special treat if you are watching your sodium intake.

MAKES 4 SERVINGS

Olive oil in a pump sprayer

1 pound large shrimp (21 to 25), peeled and deveined

6 cups seedless watermelon cubes, cut into 1-inch squares, chilled

½ medium red onion, cut into thin half-moons

24 large basil leaves, cut into thin shreds (¼ cup packed)

1 recipe Lime Vinaigrette (page 73)

Spray a large nonstick skillet with oil and heat over medium-high heat. Add the shrimp and cook, stirring occasionally, until opaque throughout, about 3 minutes. Transfer to a plate and let cool. Cover and refrigerate until chilled, at least 1 hour.

In a large serving bowl, mix the watermelon, onion, and basil. Add the shrimp and vinaigrette and toss gently. Serve chilled.

NUTRITIONAL ANALYSIS

(1 serving) 234 calories, 17 g protein, 23 g carbohydrates, 9 g fat, 2 g fiber, 143 mg cholesterol, 696 mg sodium, 466 mg potassium. Food groups: 2½ ounces meat, 1½ fruits, 1 fat.

Tuna and Vegetable Salad

Too often, tuna salad is nothing but tuna and loads of mayo. This recipe is crunchy with carrots and celery and has just enough light mayonnaise to hold it together, making it a versatile ingredient in sandwiches and with mixed greens to become a main-course salad. Use this tuna salad when you want an almost traditional sandwich filling.

MAKES 2 SERVINGS

1 (5-ounce) can low-sodium tuna in water, drained

2 small celery ribs, finely diced

1 small carrot, shredded

1 small scallion, white part only, finely chopped

2 tablespoons light mayonnaise

2 teaspoons chopped fresh parsley or dill (optional)

In a small bowl, mix all of the ingredients, including the parsley, if using. (The salad can be refrigerated in a covered container for up to 2 days.)

NUTRITIONAL ANALYSIS

(1 serving) 161 calories, 18 g protein, 6 g carbohydrates, 7 g fat, 2 g fiber, 35 mg cholesterol, 191 mg sodium, 403 mg potassium. Food groups: 2½ ounces meat, ½ vegetable.

Canned Tuna

For many years, canned tuna was notorious for its high sodium content. Now the major brands are offering reduced-sodium and even very low-sodium options, both of which may be found at your supermarket. With some searching, you should even be able to find no-salt-added tuna (Trader Joe's canned albacore tuna has gained many fans). If you are faced with regular canned tuna, place it in a sieve and rinse well under gently running cold water for a minute or so to reduce the sodium content by about 75 percent.

Tuna and White Bean Salad

In Italy, you may find the tuna and bean component served as part of an antipasti platter, but it really shines when it is expanded with greens and vegetables to make a meal. And this recipe is especially rich in beans, making it a great source of soluble fiber to help lower cholesterol.

MAKES 2 SERVINGS

2 tablespoons red wine vinegar

1 tablespoon water

1 small clove garlic, crushed through a press

¼ teaspoon dried oregano

¼ teaspoon kosher salt

¼ teaspoon crushed hot red pepper

1 tablespoon olive oil

1 (15-ounce) can no-salt-added cannellini beans, drained and rinsed

1 (5-ounce) can very low-sodium tuna in water, drained

1 medium red bell pepper, roasted, seeded, and diced (see "Roasting Red Peppers," opposite)

2 tablespoons finely chopped fresh parsley (optional)

2 cups (2 ounces) mixed salad greens

Lemon wedges, for serving

In a medium bowl, whisk together the vinegar, water, garlic, oregano, salt, and hot pepper. Whisk in the oil. Add the beans, tuna, red bell pepper, and parsley (if using) and mix well. This salad can be refrigerated in a covered container for up to 2 days.

For each serving, put 1 cup of salad greens in a wide bowl. Top with half of the tuna and bean mixture. Serve immediately with the lemon wedges for squeezing the juice onto the salad.

NUTRITIONAL ANALYSIS
(1 serving) 402 calories, 32 g protein, 52 g carbohydrates, 8 g fat, 13 g fiber, 31 mg cholesterol, 314 mg sodium, 1,282 mg potassium. Food groups: 2½ ounces meat, 2½ beans.

Roasting Red Peppers

Red bell peppers have a high flavor profile in their raw state, but roasting softens the flesh, condenses the juices, and loosens the bitter skin for easy peeling. (The skin on green peppers is too thin for roasting.) The best way to roast peppers is in the broiler. And although many cooks use a whole pepper, it is much quicker and easier to cut the pepper first into a long strip so it doesn't have to be turned.

Cut off the top "lid" and bottom inch of the pepper. Poke the stem out of the lid and discard, then set aside the top and bottom pieces. Slice the pepper vertically down the side and open it up into a long strip. Cut out the ribs and seeds. Position a broiler rack about 6 inches from the source of heat and preheat the broiler. Place the pepper strip top and bottom on the rack, skin side up. Broil until the skin is blackened and blistered, 5 minutes or longer, depending on the heat of the broiler. Let cool for a few minutes, then peel off the blackened skin. (It is not necessary to put the peppers in a bowl and cover with plastic wrap; this creates steam that softens the peppers too much.) Try not to rinse the peppers under cold water unless necessary, as the water rinses away the flavor.

Arugula, Peach, and Almond Salad

Make this salad in the summer when peaches and arugula are in season and at their best. Cling peaches (you will have to cut away the flesh from the pit) arrive first in late spring, and the freestones (with loose pits) show up throughout the summer. Nectarines are delicious in this salad, too. The combination of spicy arugula and sweet peaches will have you going back for more.   MAKES 4 SERVINGS

1 tablespoon balsamic vinegar

1 tablespoon olive oil, preferably extra-virgin

1 tablespoon water

Pinch of kosher salt

6 cups (5 ounces) baby arugula, well washed and dried

3 ripe peaches, pitted and sliced

½ cup sliced natural almonds, toasted (see "Toasting Nuts," below)

Freshly ground black pepper

In a large bowl, whisk together the vinegar, oil, water, and salt. Add the arugula, peaches, and almonds and toss. Season with the pepper. Serve immediately.

NUTRITIONAL ANALYSIS
(1 serving) 152 calories, 4 g protein, 15 g carbohydrates, 10 g fat, 4 g fiber, 0 mg cholesterol, 72 mg sodium, 431 mg potassium. Food groups: 1 vegetable, 1 fruit, ½ nuts, 1 fat.

Toasting Nuts

Nuts are valuable for adding crunch, flavor, and protein to meals, especially in salads. Toasting nuts makes a good thing better. Although nuts can be toasted in a skillet, you will get more even coloring by baking. You can use a regular oven or, to avoid heating up the kitchen, a toaster oven.

Spread the nuts on a baking sheet (or a toaster oven tray). Bake in a preheated 350°F oven (or toaster oven), stirring occasionally, until lightly browned and fragrant, about 10 minutes. Transfer to a plate and let cool.

For hazelnuts, bake until the skins are cracked, about 10 minutes. Wrap the hazelnuts in a kitchen towel and let stand about 10 minutes to cool slightly. Rub the hazelnuts in the towel to remove as much of the skins as possible. (Don't worry if a few skins remain on the nuts.)

Roasted Beet Salad with Yogurt-Dill Dressing

For years, beets were cooked by boiling, which doesn't do much for their flavor. Roasting, however, brings out their sweetness, which is balanced here with a tangy yogurt-dill dressing. This recipe keeps well in the refrigerator, so you can have it ready to serve as a cool salad or side dish.

MAKES 4 SERVINGS

1½ pounds beets (6 medium) without leaves or stems, scrubbed but unpeeled

½ cup plain nonfat yogurt

1 tablespoon cider vinegar

1 tablespoon finely chopped fresh dill, tarragon, or parsley

½ teaspoon kosher salt

¼ teaspoon freshly ground black pepper

1 clove garlic, crushed through a press

1 cup halved grape tomatoes

2 scallions, white and green parts, trimmed and thinly sliced

Preheat the oven to 400°F. Wrap each beet in aluminum foil.

Place on a rimmed baking sheet and roast until tender, about 1¼ hour, depending on the size and age of the beets. Unwrap and let cool until easy to handle. Peel the beets and cut into ½-inch-thick wedges.

In a medium bowl, whisk together the yogurt, vinegar, dill, salt, pepper, and garlic. Add the tomatoes, beets, and scallions and toss to coat. Cover and refrigerate until chilled, at least 1 hour and up to 12 hours. Serve chilled.

NUTRITIONAL ANALYSIS

(1 serving) 83 calories, 4 g protein, 17 g carbohydrates, 0 g fat, 4 g fiber, 0 mg cholesterol, 325 mg sodium, 617 mg potassium. Food groups: 2 vegetables.

Roasting Beets

Uncooked beets can be stored in the refrigerator for about a week. Get in the habit of cooking them when the oven is already on. Just wrap the beets in foil and bake directly on a baking sheet. Don't worry about the oven temperature. If the other food is cooking at the common temperature of 350°F, use it for cooking the beets, too. When the other food is removed from the oven, increase the temperature to 400°F and roast until the beets are tender. Some people like to microwave beets in a baking dish with a little water, which is a time-saver, but nothing brings out the beets' sweetness like the dry heat of an oven.

Apple Coleslaw with Buttermilk Dressing

Coleslaw is a cookout staple, but this one has a few twists to make a healthier version. Shredded apple gives it just the right amount of sweetness, and the dressing uses buttermilk as its base.

MAKES 4 SERVINGS

1 (14-ounce) bag shredded coleslaw mix

1 large red bell pepper, cored and thinly sliced (a food processor with the slicing blade does the best job)

1 Granny Smith apple, unpeeled, shredded down to the core on the large holes of a box grater

2 scallions, white and green parts, finely chopped

1 tablespoon cider vinegar

⅓ cup plus 1 tablespoon buttermilk

3 tablespoons light mayonnaise

¼ teaspoon kosher salt

½ teaspoon celery seed (optional)

¼ teaspoon freshly ground black pepper

Combine the coleslaw mix, bell pepper, apple, and scallions in a large bowl. Sprinkle with the vinegar and toss well.

In a small bowl, whisk together the buttermilk, mayonnaise, salt, celery seed (if using), and pepper. Pour over the cabbage mixture and mix well. Cover and refrigerate for at least 1 hour and up to 1 day. Serve chilled.

NUTRITIONAL ANALYSIS
(1 serving) 113 calories, 3 g protein, 17 g carbohydrates, 4 g fat, 5 g fiber, 5 mg cholesterol, 157 mg sodium, 373 mg potassium. Food groups: 1 vegetable, ½ fruit.

Asian Slaw with Ginger Dressing

This slightly spicy slaw is bound to become a favorite, as it brings lots of flavor to the table without much effort, especially if you use a food processor to prepare the cabbage, bell pepper, and carrots. Served soon after mixing, it retains its crunch; if allowed to stand more than a couple of hours, it softens, but it is still delicious.   MAKES 4 SERVINGS

1 (3-inch-long) piece of unpeeled fresh ginger, shredded on the large holes of a box grater

2 tablespoons unseasoned rice vinegar

1 clove garlic, crushed through a press

½ teaspoon kosher salt

¼ teaspoon crushed hot red pepper

1 tablespoon Asian dark sesame oil

1 tablespoon canola oil

4 cups thinly sliced Napa cabbage (about ½ small head)

1 red bell pepper, cored and cut into ¼-inch-wide strips

2 carrots, shredded

2 scallions, white and green parts, thinly sliced

2 tablespoons chopped fresh cilantro (optional)

¼ cup coarsely chopped dry-roasted unsalted peanuts

Squeeze the shredded ginger into a large bowl to extract its juice. You should have about 2 tablespoons ginger juice. Whisk in the rice vinegar, garlic, salt, and hot pepper. Gradually whisk in the sesame and canola oils.

Add the cabbage, bell pepper, carrots, scallions, and cilantro (if using) and mix well. Sprinkle with the peanuts and serve immediately. (The salad can be covered and refrigerated for 1 day. Reseason with more vinegar and sesame oil before serving.) Serve immediately or cover with plastic wrap and refrigerate.

NUTRITIONAL ANALYSIS
(1 serving) 137 calories, 4 g protein, 14 g carbohydrates, 8 g fat, 4 g fiber, 0 mg cholesterol, 290 mg sodium, 516 mg potassium. Food groups: 1½ vegetables, ½ nuts, 1 fat.

Crunchy Broccoli Slaw

Everyone knows cabbage slaw, but have you tried the broccoli slaw now available in super-market produce refrigerators? It is surprisingly versatile and makes a terrific salad.

MAKES 6 SERVINGS

½ cup dried cranberries

1 (12-ounce) bag broccoli slaw

2 scallions, white and green parts, finely chopped

¼ cup sliced natural almonds, toasted (see "Toasting Nuts," page 60)

¼ cup nonfat sour cream

2 tablespoons cider vinegar

½ teaspoon kosher salt

¼ teaspoon freshly ground black pepper

Cover the cranberries with hot tap water in a small bowl and let stand until softened, about 30 minutes. (Or place the cranberries and water in a microwave-safe bowl and microwave for 1½ minutes on high power.) Drain and pat dry.

In a medium bowl, combine the broccoli slaw, scallions, drained cranberries, almonds, sour cream, vinegar, salt, and pepper. Mix well to distribute the sour cream.

Cover with plastic wrap and refrigerate until the slaw is chilled and slightly wilted, about 1 hour and up to 12 hours. Serve chilled.

NUTRITIONAL ANALYSIS
(1 serving) 83 calories, 2 g protein, 15 g carbohydrates, 2 g fat, 3 g fiber, 0 mg cholesterol, 190 mg sodium, 75 mg potassium. Food groups: 3 vegetables.

Chopped Greek Salad

The bright colors of Greek salad are as appetizing as its flavor. Usually it is made with feta cheese, but low-sodium feta is impossible to find. However, goat cheese has a similar flavor and has a naturally low-sodium content. If you can find it, low-fat goat cheese has the least amount of sodium and fat. You can refrigerate the salad, without the cheese, for a few hours, but drain it before serving and add the goat cheese at the last minute. This is a perfect salad to serve with the Grilled Pork and Vegetable Souvlaki with Oregano-Lemon Marinade on page 97.   MAKES 4 SERVINGS

1 small red onion, cut into very thin half-moons

1 tablespoon red wine vinegar

1 tablespoon water

1 teaspoon dried oregano

1 clove garlic, minced

⅛ teaspoon freshly ground black pepper

1 tablespoon extra-virgin olive oil

1 pint grape tomatoes, cut in halves

1 medium cucumber, peeled, halved lengthwise, seeded, and cut into thin half-moons

½ cup diced (½-inch) green bell pepper

2 ounces (½ cup) crumbled regular rindless goat cheese

Soak the red onion in a small bowl of cold water for 30 minutes; drain and pat dry. (This step is optional, but it helps mellow the onion's strong flavor.)

In a large bowl, whisk together the vinegar, water, oregano, garlic, and pepper. Gradually whisk in the oil. Add the drained onion, tomatoes, cucumber, and bell pepper and toss well. Sprinkle with the goat cheese and serve at once.

NUTRITIONAL ANALYSIS

(1 serving) 95 calories, 5 g protein, 10 g carbohydrates, 5 g fat, 3 g fiber, 11 mg cholesterol, 81 mg sodium, 383 mg potassium. Food groups: 2 vegetables, ¼ dairy.

Variation

You could also make this salad with regular feta cheese in place of the goat cheese.

NUTRITIONAL ANALYSIS

(1 serving) 80 calories, 4 g protein, 10 g carbohydrates, 3 g fat, 3 g fiber, 13 mg cholesterol, 166 mg sodium, 370 mg potassium. Food groups: 2 vegetables, ¼ dairy.

Iceberg Lettuce Wedge with Russian Dressing

Poor iceberg lettuce...it doesn't get any respect. It has been shunned for prettier boutique greens and also because people think it doesn't have any health benefits. This is not true, for iceberg is more filling than more delicate lettuces, and it is also a good source of potassium. It is sturdy enough to stand up to thick salad dressings, as you can see here, in this steakhouse-style side dish.   MAKES 2 SERVINGS

½ head iceberg lettuce, cut in half lengthwise to make 2 wedges

½ cup halved grape tomatoes

½ medium cucumber, peeled and thinly sliced

½ small sweet onion, cut into thin half-moons

1 recipe Russian Dressing (page 74)

For each serving, put an iceberg wedge on a serving plate and surround with the tomatoes, cucumber, and onion. Top each wedge with the dressing and serve.

NUTRITIONAL ANALYSIS

(1 serving) 194 calories, 4 g protein, 22 mg carbohydrates, 11 g fat, 3 g fiber, 12 mg cholesterol, 318 mg sodium, 444 mg potassium. Food groups: 2 vegetables, 2 fats.

Kale, Pear, and Bulgur Salad

Kale is not a tender green, but when it is massaged with lemon juice, it softens enough to be served as a salad. Kale's natural bitterness is mellowed here with sweet pears, and crunchy walnuts do their part to make this a very interesting and tasty salad. Add roasted salmon to turn this into a main course. MAKES 4 SERVINGS

½ cup bulgur

1¾ cups boiling water

8 ounces curly kale

2 tablespoons fresh lemon juice

½ teaspoon kosher salt

2 ripe pears, such as Anjou or Comice, cored and thinly sliced

½ cup walnut pieces, toasted (see "Toasting Nuts," page 60) and coarsely chopped

2 tablespoons extra-virgin olive oil

Freshly ground black pepper

Put the bulgur in a medium heatproof bowl and add the boiling water. Let stand until the bulgur is tender, about 30 minutes. Drain in a wire sieve. Press the excess liquid from the bulgur. Set aside.

Pull off and discard the thick stems from the kale. Taking a few pieces at a time, stack the kale and coarsely slice crosswise into ½-inch-thick strips. Transfer to a large bowl of cold water and agitate to loosen any grit. Lift the kale out of the water, leaving any dirt behind in the water. Dry the kale in a salad spinner or pat dry with paper towels.

Sprinkle the kale with the lemon juice and salt. Using your hands, rub the kale until softened, about 2 minutes. Fluff the bulgur with a fork and add to the kale with the pears and walnuts. Drizzle with the oil and toss. Season with the pepper. Serve at once or refrigerate for up to 2 hours.

NUTRITIONAL ANALYSIS
(1 serving) 295 calories, 8 g protein, 34 g carbohydrates, 17 g fat, 8 g fiber, 0 mg cholesterol, 278 mg sodium, 516 mg potassium. Food groups: ¼ whole grain, 2 vegetables, 1 fruit, ½ nuts, 1 fat.

Potato Salad with Asparagus and Peas

Potatoes are a good match for many ingredients, and there is no reason your potato salad shouldn't feature other vegetables to keep it from being too starchy. Yogurt perks up the standard dressing.   MAKES 10 SERVINGS

3 large red-skinned potatoes (1½ pounds), scrubbed but unpeeled

8 ounces asparagus, woody stems discarded, cut into 1-inch lengths

2 tablespoons white wine or cider vinegar

3 celery ribs, thinly sliced

½ cup thawed frozen peas

2 scallions, white and green parts, finely chopped

2 tablespoons finely chopped fresh parsley

¼ cup plain low-fat yogurt

2 tablespoons light mayonnaise

½ teaspoon kosher salt

¼ teaspoon freshly ground black pepper

Put the potatoes in a large saucepan and add enough cold water to cover by 1 inch. Cover and bring to a boil over high heat. Set the lid ajar and reduce the heat to medium-low. Cook until the potatoes are tender when pierced with the tip of a sharp knife, about 30 minutes. Using a slotted spoon, transfer the potatoes to a colander; keep the water boiling. Rinse the potatoes under cold running water. Transfer to a chopping board and let stand until cool enough to handle.

Meanwhile, add the asparagus to the boiling water and cook just until tender, about 5 minutes. Drain in the colander, rinse under cold running water, and pat dry with paper towels.

Cut each potato in half and then into ½-inch-thick slices. Transfer to a medium bowl and sprinkle the warm potatoes with the vinegar. Add the asparagus, celery, peas, scallions, and parsley. In a small bowl, whisk together the yogurt, mayonnaise, salt, and pepper. Pour over the potato mixture and mix gently. Cover with plastic wrap and refrigerate until chilled, at least 1 hour, or up to 2 days. Serve chilled.

NUTRITIONAL ANALYSIS
(1 serving) 75 calories, 3 g protein, 14 g carbohydrates, 1 g fat, 2 g fiber, 1 mg cholesterol, 154 mg sodium, 426 mg potassium. Food groups: 1 starchy vegetable.

Lentil and Goat Cheese Salad

This hearty salad is especially good when made with green (also called Puy) lentils, which are more attractive than common brown lentils, but they both work well. Just be careful not to overcook them. If you make the salad more than a few hours ahead, it will probably need reseasoning with vinegar before serving.   MAKES 6 SERVINGS

1 cup green (Puy) or brown lentils

2 tablespoons sherry or cider vinegar

2 tablespoons water

Freshly grated zest of 1 lemon

½ teaspoon kosher salt

¼ teaspoon freshly ground black pepper

2 tablespoons olive oil, preferably extra-virgin

1 medium red bell pepper, cored and cut into ¼-inch dice

2 celery ribs, cut into ¼-inch dice

1 medium carrot, peeled and cut into ¼-inch dice

2 tablespoons finely chopped fresh basil, oregano, or parsley

4 ounces (1 cup) crumbled goat cheese

Bring a medium saucepan of water to a boil over high heat. Add the lentils and cook (just like pasta) until tender, about 30 minutes. Drain in a wire sieve, rinse under cold running water, and drain well.

In a large bowl, whisk together the vinegar, water, lemon zest, salt, and pepper. Gradually whisk in the oil.

Add the lentils, bell pepper, celery, carrot, and basil and toss well. (The salad can be covered and refrigerated for up to 1 day.) Sprinkle with the goat cheese and serve chilled or at room temperature.

NUTRITIONAL ANALYSIS

(1 serving) 170 calories, 9 g protein, 22 g carbohydrates, 5 g fat, 11 g fiber, 0 mg cholesterol, 21 mg sodium, 428 mg potassium. Food groups: 1 beans, 1 vegetable, 1 dairy, 1 fat.

Weeknight Tossed Green Salad

To help you calculate calories and other nutritional information in a big salad, here is one with the basic ingredients—greens, tomatoes, cucumbers, and a handful of nuts. Salad greens come in convenient premeasured bags (although they do need to be rinsed before using), or you can substitute 6 loosely packed cups of your favorite lettuces. Remember that colorful greens have the most nutrients. Add any of your favorite salad dressings in this book for low-fat options.   MAKES 4 SERVINGS

---

1 (5-ounce bag) mixed
salad greens

1 cup halved grape
tomatoes

1 cucumber, peeled,
seeded, and sliced

½ cup sunflower or
pumpkin seeds or sliced
natural almonds

American-Style French
Dressing, Lemon
Vinaigrette, Mustard
Vinaigrette, Creamy
Ranch Dressing, or
Russian Dressing
(pages 72 to 74)

Toss the salad greens, tomatoes, and cucumber together in a large bowl. Sprinkle with the seeds. Drizzle with the dressing and toss again. Serve immediately.

NUTRITIONAL ANALYSIS
(1 serving without dressing) 89 calories, 4 g protein, 7 g carbohydrates, 6 g fat, 3 g fiber, 0 mg cholesterol, 10 mg sodium, 389 mg potassium. Food groups: 2 vegetables, ½ nuts.

Baby Spinach and Strawberry Salad

I'm giving the recipe for this delicious, naturally sweet salad without any protein so it can be served as a side salad for dinner. However, with the addition of some goat cheese or sliced chicken breast, it is easily transformed into a main-course salad.

MAKES 4 SERVINGS

1 pound fresh strawberries, hulled

2 tablespoons balsamic vinegar

2 tablespoons olive oil, preferably extra-virgin

2 tablespoons water

Pinch of kosher salt

Pinch of freshly ground black pepper

2 teaspoons poppy seeds

7½ cups (6 ounces) baby spinach

½ cup toasted, skinned, and coarsely chopped hazelnuts (see "Toasting Nuts," page 60)

4 ounces (1 cup) crumbled goat cheese (optional)

Coarsely chop ¼ cup of the strawberries and transfer to a blender. Slice the remaining strawberries and set aside.

In the blender, puree the chopped strawberries, vinegar, oil, water, salt, and pepper until smooth. Add the poppy seeds and pulse once or twice just to combine.

Toss the baby spinach and strawberry dressing in a large bowl. Add the hazelnuts and reserved sliced strawberries and toss again. Sprinkle with the goat cheese, if using. Serve at once.

NUTRITIONAL ANALYSIS

(1 serving with optional goat cheese) 211 calories, 4 g protein, 14 g carbohydrates, 16 g fat, 5 g fiber, 0 mg cholesterol, 85 mg sodium, 291 mg potassium. Food groups: 1 vegetable, 1 fruit, ½ nuts, 1 fat, 1 dairy.

Salad Dressings

Salad dressings can be the downfall of many a well-intentioned diet plan. Here is a collection of homemade reduced-fat, low-calorie dressings that I guarantee are better than any commercial brand in a bottle. All of these dressings can be refrigerated in a covered container for at least 3 days. Whisk them well before serving.

American-Style French Dressing

If you like thick, red "French" dressing, this one's for you. (There really isn't anything French about it, so how it got its name is a mystery.) It is best served over sturdy greens such as romaine lettuce.

MAKES ABOUT ¾ CUP

¼ cup no-salt-added tomato ketchup

2 tablespoons minced shallot

2 tablespoons water

1 tablespoon cider vinegar

1 clove garlic, crushed through a press

¼ teaspoon freshly ground black pepper

2 tablespoons canola oil

In a small bowl, whisk together the ketchup, shallot, water, vinegar, garlic, and pepper. Gradually whisk in the oil.

NUTRITIONAL ANALYSIS
(1 serving: 2 tablespoons) 90 calories, 0 g protein, 7 g carbohydrates, 7 g fat, 0 g fiber, 0 mg cholesterol, 1 mg sodium, 24 mg potassium. Food groups: 1 fat.

Asian Ginger Dressing

This dressing has just enough soy sauce to give it an Asian flavor.

MAKES ABOUT ½ CUP

1 (3-inch) piece fresh ginger, unpeeled and shredded on the large holes of a box grater

2 tablespoons rice vinegar

1 tablespoon low-sodium soy sauce

1 tablespoon plus 1 teaspoon water

¼ teaspoon crushed hot red pepper

¼ teaspoon amber agave nectar

1 tablespoon vegetable oil

1 tablespoon Asian dark sesame oil

Squeeze the shredded ginger in your hand and extract the juice into a medium bowl; you should have about 2 teaspoons. (Or put the ginger in a wire sieve and press hard with a wooden spoon to extract the juice.) Add the vinegar, soy sauce, water, hot pepper, and agave and whisk well. Gradually whisk in the vegetable and sesame oils.

NUTRITIONAL ANALYSIS
(1 serving: 2 tablespoons) 71 calories, 0 g protein, 2 g carbohydrates, 7 g fat, 0 g fiber, 0 mg cholesterol, 151 mg sodium, 27 mg potassium. Food groups: 1 fat.

Lemon Vinaigrette

Lemon is well known for its ability to enliven the taste of food. This vinaigrette can be used to dress green and even fruit salads, but also try it as a condiment for grilled fish and chicken. The lime variation is useful, too, especially with spicy foods.

MAKES ABOUT ½ CUP

Freshly grated zest of 1 lemon

3 tablespoons fresh lemon juice

3 tablespoons water

Pinch of kosher salt

Pinch of freshly ground black pepper

2 tablespoons olive oil, preferably
    extra-virgin

In a small bowl, whisk together the lemon zest and juice, water, salt, and pepper. Gradually whisk in the oil. (Or combine all of the ingredients in a small jar and shake well to blend.)

NUTRITIONAL ANALYSIS
(1 serving: 2 tablespoons) 64 calories, 0 g protein, 1 g carbohydrates, 7 g fat, 1 g fiber, 0 mg cholesterol, 50 mg sodium, 16 mg potassium. Food groups: 1 fat.

Lime Vinaigrette

Substitute lime zest and juice for the lemon zest and juice.

NUTRITIONAL ANALYSIS
(1 serving: 2 tablespoons) 64 calories, 0 g protein, 1 g carbohydrates, 7 g fat, 1 g fiber, 0 mg cholesterol, 50 mg sodium, 16 mg potassium. Food groups: 1 fat.

Mustard Vinaigrette

Don't be surprised if this becomes your house dressing. If you wish, add a small garlic clove, crushed through a press.

MAKES ½ CUP

2 tablespoons red wine vinegar

2 tablespoons olive oil, preferably
    extra-virgin

2 tablespoons plain low-fat yogurt

2 tablespoons water

1 teaspoon Dijon mustard

¼ teaspoon kosher salt

¼ teaspoon freshly ground black pepper

In a small bowl, whisk together all of the ingredients. (Or combine all of the ingredients in a small jar with a tight-fitting lid and shake well.)

NUTRITIONAL ANALYSIS
(1 serving: 2 tablespoons) 67 calories, 0 g protein, 0 g carbohydrates, 7 g fat, 0 g fiber, 0 mg cholesterol, 282 mg sodium, 21 mg potassium. Food groups: 1 fat.

Creamy Ranch Dressing

Commercial thick and creamy dressings can ruin the nutritional value of a green salad. Not this one, which uses buttermilk and light mayonnaise as its base.

MAKES ABOUT ¾ CUP

⅓ cup plus 1 tablespoon buttermilk

¼ cup light mayonnaise

1 scallion, white and green parts, minced

2 tablespoons cider vinegar

½ teaspoon celery seed

¼ teaspoon freshly ground black pepper

In a small bowl, whisk together all of the ingredients.

NUTRITIONAL ANALYSIS
(1 serving: 2 tablespoons) 42 calories, 1 g protein, 2 g carbohydrates, 4 g fat, 0 g fiber, 4 mg cholesterol, 85 mg sodium, 43 mg potassium. Food groups: 1 fat.

Russian Dressing

For a change of pace from mixed greens and vinaigrette, dive into this thick dressing, poured over cool and crunchy iceberg lettuce.

MAKES ⅔ CUP

¼ cup plain low-fat yogurt

¼ cup light mayonnaise

2 tablespoons no-salt-added tomato ketchup

1 tablespoon reduced-sodium sweet pickle relish

½ teaspoon Worcestershire sauce

⅛ teaspoon hot red pepper sauce

In a small bowl, whisk together all of the ingredients.

NUTRITIONAL ANALYSIS
(1 serving: 2 tablespoons) 64 calories, 1 g protein, 6 g carbohydrates, 4 g fat, 0 g fiber, 5 mg cholesterol, 96 mg sodium, 41 mg potassium. Food groups: 1 fat.

Beef, Pork, and Lamb

Red meat can play a role in a healthy diet. It is just a matter of choosing lean cuts and exercising portion control. Many people grill steaks and chops, a cooking method that does not call for added fat, and then top them with a fatty sauce. I often prefer to cook the meat in a nonstick skillet to create flavorful pan juices that can be used to make a terrific pan sauce. Augment the meat with lots of vegetables, and you will have a meal in a skillet that needs very little to round it out. So here are my favorite recipes for beef, pork, and lamb, cooked the DASH way.

Curry-Rubbed Sirloin with Peanut Dipping Sauce

Many cooks like to marinate meat before cooking, but it takes time for the liquid to transfer flavor to the food. Rubs work immediately and are real time-savers. This Southeast Asian–inspired dish can be served with brown rice and a vegetable stir-fry. Leftover peanut dip can be served with raw vegetables at another meal. **MAKES 8 SERVINGS**

Sirloin

1 teaspoon curry powder

½ teaspoon ground ginger

½ teaspoon granulated garlic

½ teaspoon kosher salt

½ teaspoon freshly ground black pepper

Canola oil in a spray pump

1¾ pounds sirloin steak, about 1 inch thick, excess fat trimmed

Peanut Dipping Sauce

¼ cup smooth peanut butter

3 tablespoons brewed cold black tea

3 tablespoons light coconut milk

2 teaspoons peeled and minced fresh ginger

2 teaspoons reduced-sodium soy sauce

1½ teaspoons rice vinegar

2 teaspoons curry powder

1 clove garlic, crushed through a press

Chopped fresh cilantro or mint, for garnish

To prepare the sirloin: In a small bowl, mix the curry powder, ground ginger, granulated garlic, salt, and pepper. Spray the oil on both sides of the steak and season with the curry mixture. Let stand at room temperature while making the peanut sauce.

To make the Peanut Dipping Sauce: In a medium bowl, whisk together the peanut butter, tea, coconut milk, ginger, soy sauce, vinegar, curry, and garlic.

Position a broiler rack about 4 inches from the source of heat and preheat on high. Oil the broiler rack and add the steak. Broil, flipping the steak over after 3 minutes, until browned on both sides and the meat feels only slightly resilient when pressed in the center, about 6 minutes for medium-rare. Transfer to a carving board and let stand for 3 minutes.

Pour the peanut sauce into eight ramekins. Carve the steak across the grain into ½-inch-thick slices. Transfer to a platter and sprinkle with the cilantro. Serve hot, with the peanut sauce.

NUTRITIONAL ANALYSIS
(1 [4-ounce] serving) 236 calories, 28 g protein, 0 g carbohydrates, 12 g fat, 0 g fiber, 100 mg cholesterol, 191 mg sodium, 439 mg potassium. Food groups: 4 ounces meat.

(1 [3-ounce] serving) 189 calories, 23 g protein, 0 g carbohydrates, 10 g fat, 0 g fiber, 80 mg cholesterol, 153 mg sodium, 343 mg potassium. Food groups: 3 ounces meat.

(1 serving, Peanut Dipping Sauce: 3 tablespoons) 198 calories, 4 g protein, 10 g carbohydrates, 9 g fat, 1 g fiber, 0 mg cholesterol, 159 mg sodium, 157 mg potassium. Food groups: 1 nut.

Meat Temperatures

An instant-read thermometer is a reliable tool, but it works best with roasts and large cuts of meat that will support the thin probe. For thin cuts of meat such as chops and steaks and for boneless chicken breast, it is best to rely on "the touch test." As meat cooks, its liquid evaporates and the flesh becomes firmer. Press the meat with a forefinger to determine its doneness. In general, rare meat feels soft, medium is slightly resilient, and well-done is firm. Or use a small, sharp knife and check the internal color of the meat.

Sirloin, Shiitake, and Asparagus Stir-Fry

Stir-fries allow the DASH-centric cook to use a reasonable amount of meat with lots of vegetables. Serve with ½ cup of Basic Brown Rice (page 174), if you wish. If you care to sprinkle soy sauce on your serving, use a very light hand.　　　MAKES 6 SERVINGS

Sauce

¾ cup Homemade Chicken Broth (page 38) or canned low-sodium chicken broth

2 tablespoons dry sherry or dry vermouth

1 tablespoon rice vinegar

1 tablespoon low-sodium soy sauce

1 tablespoon cornstarch

½ teaspoon freshly ground black pepper

Stir-Fry

4 teaspoons canola oil

1 pound sirloin steak, excess fat trimmed, cut across the grain into ¼-inch-thick slices and then into 2-inch strips

1 tablespoon peeled and minced fresh ginger

2 cloves garlic, minced

12 ounces thin asparagus, woody stems discarded, cut into 1-inch lengths

6 ounces shiitake mushroom caps, sliced

6 ounces sugar snap or snow peas, trimmed

½ cup water

3 scallions, white and green parts, cut into 1-inch lengths

To make the sauce: In a small bowl, whisk together the broth, sherry, vinegar, soy sauce, cornstarch, and pepper.

To make the stir-fry: Heat 2 teaspoons of the oil in a large nonstick skillet or wok over medium-high heat. In two batches, add the steak and cook, stirring occasionally, until seared, about 2 minutes. Transfer to a plate.

Heat the remaining 2 teaspoons oil in the skillet over medium-high heat. Add the ginger and garlic and stir until fragrant, about 30 seconds. Add the asparagus, shiitake, and sugar snap peas and stir well. Add the water and cook, stirring often, until the water has evaporated and the vegetables are crisp-tender, about 3 minutes. During the last minute, stir in the scallions.

Add the sauce mixture to the skillet and stir until thickened and boiling, about 30 seconds. Return the steak to the skillet and stir well. Transfer to a serving platter. Serve hot.

NUTRITIONAL ANALYSIS
(1 serving) 182 calories, 20 g protein, 10 g carbohydrates, 7 g fat, 3 g fiber, 45 mg cholesterol, 157 mg sodium, 584 mg potassium. Food groups: 3 ounces meat, 2 vegetables.

Beef and Mushrooms with Sour Cream–Dill Sauce

Beef Stroganoff can be an excessively rich dish. I've reduced the guilt factor by using lean sirloin, lots of mushrooms, and reduced-fat sour cream. Broccoli Ziti (page 162) would be a good match for a side dish. MAKES 4 SERVINGS

2 teaspoons canola oil, plus more in a pump sprayer

1 pound sirloin steak, excess fat trimmed, cut across the grain in ½-inch-thick slices and then into 2-inch-wide pieces

12 ounces cremini mushrooms, sliced

¼ cup finely chopped shallots

2 teaspoons cornstarch

¾ cup Homemade Beef Stock (page 39)

½ cup reduced-fat sour cream

1 tablespoon finely chopped fresh dill

½ teaspoon kosher salt

½ teaspoon freshly ground black pepper

Spray a large nonstick skillet with oil and heat over medium-high heat. Add half of the sirloin and cook, flipping the sirloin pieces halfway through cooking, until browned on both sides, about 2 minutes. Transfer to a plate. Repeat with the remaining sirloin.

Heat the 2 teaspoons oil in the skillet over medium heat. Add the mushrooms and cook, stirring occasionally, until their liquid evaporates and they begin to brown, about 6 minutes. Stir in the shallots and cook until softened, about 1 minute.

In a small bowl, sprinkle the cornstarch over the broth and stir to dissolve. Stir into the mushrooms and cook until boiling and thickened. Stir in the sour cream, dill, salt, and pepper. Return the sirloin and any juices on the plate to the skillet and cook just until heated through, about 30 seconds. Serve hot.

NUTRITIONAL ANALYSIS
(1 serving) 275 calories, 31 g protein, 9 g carbohydrates, 13 g fat, 1 g fiber, 72 mg cholesterol, 354 mg sodium, 899 mg potassium. Food groups: 4½ ounces meat, 1 vegetable, 1 fat.

Filet Mignon *au Poivre* with Bourbon-Shallot Sauce

This variation of steak *au poivre* has an American kick from its bourbon pan sauce, although you can use the traditional brandy or Cognac. It has a spicy crust of four different peppercorns, which are sold as a blend at specialty markets and many supermarkets. If you can't find it, substitute 2 teaspoons whole peppercorns (because the red and green peppercorns reduce the pepper blend's heat, you can use more of the blended peppercorns). Serve with the Smashed Yukon Golds with Buttermilk and Scallions and Creamed Spinach with Mushrooms on pages 173 and 177 for a real steakhouse meal.   MAKES 4 SERVINGS

1 tablespoon four-peppercorn blend (a commercial blend of black, white, red, and green peppercorns)

4 (6-ounce) filets mignons

1 teaspoon canola oil, plus more in a pump sprayer

¼ cup finely chopped shallots

¼ cup bourbon, brandy, or Cognac

1 cup Homemade Beef Stock (page 39) or canned low-sodium beef broth

1 tablespoon cold unsalted butter

Pinch of kosher salt

Coarsely crush the peppercorns in a mortar and pestle or on a work surface under a heavy skillet. Spread the crushed peppercorns on a plate. Sprinkle the peppercorns evenly over both sides of the filets mignons, pressing them into the meat to adhere.

Spray enough oil in a large nonstick skillet to lightly coat the bottom, and heat over medium-high heat. Add the filets mignons and cook until the undersides are well browned, about 4 minutes. Turn and brown the other sides until the meat feels slightly resilient, about 4 minutes for medium-rare meat. Transfer to a plate.

Combine the shallots and the 1 teaspoon oil in the skillet and cook over medium heat, stirring often, until the shallots soften, about 2 minutes. Add the bourbon and cook until almost completely evaporated, about 1 minute. Add the stock and bring to a boil over high heat, scraping up the browned bits in the skillet with a wooden spatula. Boil until reduced to ½ cup, about 2 minutes. Remove from the heat and whisk in the butter and salt.

Serve each steak on a dinner plate, topped with a spoonful of sauce.

NUTRITIONAL ANALYSIS
(1 serving) 315 calories, 34 g protein, 2 g carbohydrates, 14 g fat, 0 g fiber, 104 mg cholesterol, 123 mg sodium, 440 mg potassium. Food groups: 5 ounces meat.

Spiced Roast Eye of Round

This is another recipe intended to provide leftovers for other meals—in this case, lean roast beef. The spice mixture is less assertive than you might imagine, but you can scrape it off the meat when making sandwiches and salads, if you wish. Eye of round is a very lean cut and should be roasted no more than medium-rare or it will toughen. And be sure to carve it as thinly as possible.   MAKES 12 SERVINGS

1 teaspoon cumin seeds

1 teaspoon coriander seeds

½ teaspoon whole black peppercorns

½ teaspoon kosher salt

½ teaspoon ground ginger

¼ teaspoon freshly ground black pepper

⅛ teaspoon cayenne pepper

1 (3-pound) beef eye of round roast, tied

1 clove garlic, cut into about 12 slivers

Olive oil in a pump sprayer

Position a rack in the center of the oven, and preheat the oven to 400°F.

Coarsely crush together the cumin, coriander, and peppercorns in a mortar, in an electric spice grinder, or on a work counter under a heavy skillet. Transfer to a bowl and add the salt, ginger, pepper, and cayenne.

Using the tip of a small knife, make 1-inch-deep incisions in the beef and stuff a garlic clove sliver into each slit. Spray the beef with oil and sprinkle with the spice mixture. Place the roast on a meat rack in a roasting pan.

Roast for 10 minutes. Reduce the oven temperature to 350°F and continue roasting until an instant-read thermometer inserted in the center of the beef reads 125°F for medium-rare, about 1 hour. Transfer the beef to a carving board and let stand for 10 minutes.

Remove the string and cut the meat crosswise into thin slices. Transfer to a serving platter and pour the carving juices over the beef. Serve immediately.

NUTRITIONAL ANALYSIS
(1 serving: 3 ounces) 185 calories, 33 g protein, 0 g carbohydrates, 5 g fat, 0 g fiber, 84 mg cholesterol, 125 mg sodium, 277 mg potassium. Food groups: 4½ ounces meat.

Beef Fajitas with Two Peppers

Fajitas are a real crowd-pleaser, fun to make and eat. To lighten the sodium load, serve with lettuce leaves instead of flour tortillas if you wish.　　　MAKES 6 SERVINGS

2 teaspoons olive oil, plus more in a pump sprayer

1 pound sirloin steak, excess fat trimmed, cut across the grain into ½-inch-thick slices and then into 2-inch-wide pieces

1 large red bell pepper, cored and cut into ¼-inch-wide strips

1 large green bell pepper, cored and cut into ¼-inch-wide strips

1 medium red onion, cut into thin half-moons

2 cloves garlic, minced

1 tablespoon Mexican Seasoning (page xiv)

12 (8-inch) flour tortillas or Boston lettuce leaves, for serving

Lime wedges, for serving

Spray a large nonstick skillet with oil and heat over medium-high heat. Add half of the sirloin and cook, flipping the sirloin pieces halfway through cooking, until browned on both sides, about 2 minutes. Transfer to a plate. Repeat with the remaining sirloin.

Heat the 2 teaspoons oil in the skillet over medium-high heat. Add the bell peppers, onion, and garlic. Cook, stirring occasionally, until tender, about 7 minutes. Stir in the beef with any juices and the Mexican Seasoning. Transfer to a platter.

To serve, fill a flour tortilla or lettuce leaf with the beef mixture and squeeze lime juice on top. Roll up and serve.

NUTRITIONAL ANALYSIS

(1 serving on lettuce leaves: 2 fajitas) 231 calories, 24 g protein, 6 g carbohydrates, 12 g fat, 2 g fiber, 44 mg cholesterol, 59 mg sodium, 490 mg potassium. Food groups: 3 ounces meat, 1 vegetable, 1 fat.

(1 serving on 8-inch tortillas: 2 fajitas) 377 calories, 29 g protein, 36 g carbohydrates, 13 g fat, 6 g fiber, 44 mg cholesterol, 319 mg sodium, 490 mg potassium. Food groups: 3 ounces meat, 2 whole grains, 1 vegetable, 1 fat.

Tortillas

These staples of Mexican cooking are another food category for which it is worth taking the time to check labels. Flour tortillas, even the whole-wheat variety (which carries its own health benefits over white flour tortillas), are fairly high in sodium (about 300 mg for two 8-inch tortillas). And the bigger the tortilla, the larger the sodium load, so a "burrito-size tortilla" has about 450 mg sodium. Corn tortillas have much less sodium (about 130 mg for the average 6-inch tortilla). Using large lettuce leaves (such as romaine, Boston, or Bibb) in place of tortillas will allow you to drastically cut the amount of sodium in a Mexican meal of fajitas or tacos, and increase your vegetable intake, too.

Ground Sirloin and Pinto Chili

Many a chili simmers for hours, but you may not always have the time. This version is ready in no time and is worth making in a double batch to freeze for other meals. It is on the mild side, so feel free to spice it up with the optional chipotle chili. Serve it over brown rice or whole-wheat macaroni and top it with your favorite fixings…just remember to add these to the total calorie count. This chili is very high in total fiber and rich in soluble fiber.

MAKES 6 SERVINGS

1 tablespoon olive oil

1 medium yellow onion, chopped

1 medium green bell pepper, cored and chopped

2 cloves garlic, minced

1¼ pounds ground sirloin

2 tablespoons chili powder

½ teaspoon pure ground chipotle chili, or 1 minced canned chipotle chili with its clinging adobo, or ¼ teaspoon cayenne (optional)

½ teaspoon kosher salt

1 (28-ounce) can reduced-sodium chopped tomatoes in juice, undrained

2 (15-ounce) cans reduced-sodium pinto beans, drained and well rinsed

Optional toppings: shredded low-fat Cheddar cheese, nonfat sour cream, chopped fresh cilantro leaves

Heat the oil in a large saucepan over medium heat. Add the onion and bell pepper and cook, stirring occasionally, until softened, about 3 minutes. Stir in the garlic and cook until fragrant, about 1 minute. Add the sirloin and cook, stirring often and breaking up the meat with the side of the spoon, until it loses its raw look, about 6 minutes. Stir in the chili powder, ground chipotle (if using), and salt, and cook for 1 minute, stirring often.

Stir in the tomatoes with their juice and bring to a boil over high heat. Return the heat to medium and cook at a brisk simmer, stirring occasionally, until the juices have thickened slightly, about 15 minutes. Add the beans and cook until heated through, about 5 minutes. If you like a thicker chili, mash some of the beans into the cooking liquid with a large spoon. Spoon into bowls, add the toppings if desired, and serve hot.

NUTRITIONAL ANALYSIS
(1 serving) 288 calories, 28 g protein, 24 g carbohydrates, 8 g fat, 7 g fiber, 67 mg cholesterol, 428 mg sodium, 468 mg potassium. Food groups: 3 ounces meat, 1 beans, 1½ vegetables, 1 fat.

Sirloin and Black Bean Burgers with Fresh Tomato Salsa

These thick and juicy burgers, with a nutritional profile that has been improved with the addition of fiber-rich black beans, can be grilled outdoors, if you prefer. The beans heat up in the burger and cook it from the inside out, so you won't get a rare patty. Nevertheless, it will be delicious.

MAKES 4 SERVINGS

Salsa

2 plum (Roma) tomatoes, seeded and cut into ¼-inch dice, or 1 cup coarsely chopped grape or cherry tomatoes

2 tablespoons minced white or yellow onion

1 tablespoon fresh lime juice

1 tablespoon minced fresh cilantro

1 small jalapeño or serrano chili, seeded and minced

1 clove garlic, minced

Pinch of kosher salt

Burgers

1 pound ground sirloin

1 (15-ounce) can reduced-sodium black beans, drained and rinsed

1 teaspoon chili powder

½ teaspoon kosher salt

½ teaspoon freshly ground black pepper

¼ teaspoon granulated garlic or garlic powder

¼ teaspoon granulated onion or onion powder

Olive oil in a pump sprayer

4 whole-wheat buns, toasted (optional)

2 ripe avocados, halved, pitted, peeled, and sliced

To make the salsa: In a medium serving bowl, mix together the tomatoes, onion, lime juice, cilantro, jalapeño, garlic, and salt. Set aside while making the burgers.

To make the burgers: In a medium bowl, mix together the ground sirloin, beans, chili powder, salt, pepper, granulated garlic, and granulated onion. Using hands rinsed under cold water, shape the meat mixture into four 3½-inch burgers. If the beans poke through the ground sirloin, press them back into place.

Spray a large nonstick skillet with oil and heat over medium-high heat. Add the burgers and cook, turning after 2 minutes, until browned on both sides, about 5 minutes for medium burgers. Transfer to a platter.

For each serving, place a burger on a bun, if using, and top with a spoonful of the salsa and a few avocado slices. Serve at once, with the remaining salsa on the side.

NUTRITIONAL ANALYSIS

(1 burger, without bun) 334 calories, 30 g protein, 22 g carbohydrates, 16 g fat, 10 g fiber,

70 mg cholesterol, 588 mg sodium, 1,078 mg potassium. Food groups: 3 ounces meat, 1½ beans, ½ vegetable.

(1 burger, with bun) 494 calories, 37 g protein, 53 g carbohydrates, 19 g fat, 17 g fiber, 70 mg cholesterol, 928 mg sodium, 1,232 mg potassium. Food groups: 3 ounces meat, 2 whole grains, 1½ beans, ½ vegetable.

Burger Buns

Be knowledgeable about the nutritional profile of a burger bun. The average whole-wheat hamburger bun has 160 calories, 3 g fat, and 340 mg sodium and is the equivalent of 2 servings of bread. If you are having a day where your grain and sodium intakes are light, go for it. Otherwise, skip the bun. This burger is so flavorful, you won't miss the bread.

Beef and Bulgur Meat Loaf

Many cooks think that fatty ground round or chuck is necessary to make a juicy meat loaf, but this family-friendly recipe proves that theory incorrect. The vegetables and bulgur (cracked wheat) add flavor and moisture. This could end up as your "go to" meat loaf.

MAKES 8 SERVINGS

1 cup boiling water

½ cup bulgur

2 teaspoons canola oil, plus more in a pump sprayer

1 medium yellow onion, chopped

1 medium red bell pepper, cored and cut into ¼-inch dice

2 cloves garlic, minced

¼ cup plus 2 tablespoons low-salt tomato ketchup

1 tablespoon Worcestershire sauce (see note on page 88)

1 teaspoon kosher salt

½ teaspoon freshly ground black pepper

2 large egg whites

1 pound ground sirloin

In a heatproof medium bowl, combine the boiling water and bulgur and let stand until the bulgur has softened and absorbed the water, about 20 minutes.

Meanwhile, preheat the oven to 350°F. Line a rimmed baking sheet with aluminum foil and spray with oil.

Heat the 2 teaspoons oil in a medium nonstick skillet over medium heat. Add the onion, bell pepper, and garlic and cook, stirring occasionally, until tender, about 6 minutes. Transfer to a bowl and cool slightly.

Drain the bulgur in a wire sieve, pressing hard on the bulgur to extract the excess water. Add to the bowl with the vegetables, then stir in ¼ cup of the ketchup, Worcestershire sauce, salt, and pepper. (Adding these ingredients at this point helps to cool the vegetables so the egg whites won't cook from the heat.) Stir in the egg whites. Add the ground sirloin and mix just until combined. Shape into an 8 × 4-inch loaf on the foil-lined baking sheet.

Bake until the loaf is golden brown and an instant-read thermometer inserted in the center reads 165°F, about 40 minutes. During the last 5 minutes, spread the top of the loaf with the 2 tablespoons ketchup.

Let stand for 10 minutes. Slice and serve hot.

NUTRITIONAL ANALYSIS

(1 serving: ⅛ loaf) 162 calories, 15 g protein, 16 g carbohydrates, 4 g fat, 3 g fiber, 35 mg cholesterol, 322 mg sodium, 351 mg potassium. Food groups: 1 whole grain, 2 ounces meat, ½ vegetable.

NOTE: Worcestershire sauce is also available in a reduced-sodium version. However, the reduction is only about 10 mg per teaspoon, so in the long run it may not be worth the effort it takes to find it. (The last time I looked for it, I had to go to four supermarkets before I found a bottle.)

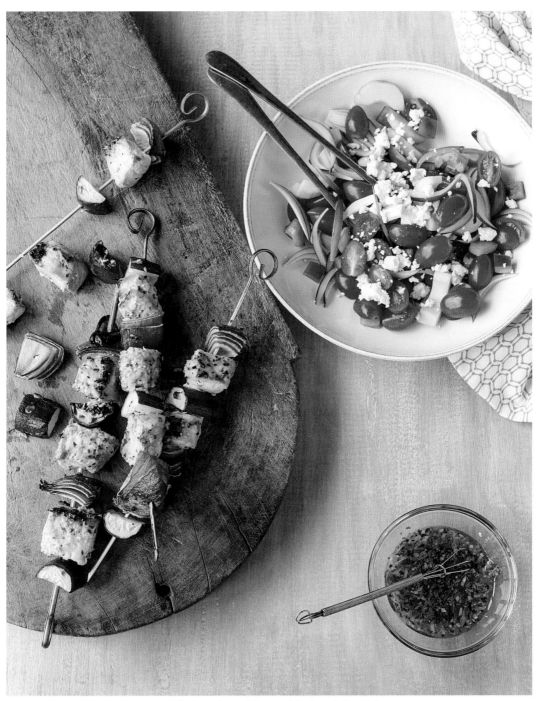

Grilled Pork and Vegetable Souvlaki with
Oregano-Lemon Marinade, page 97;
Chopped Greek Salad, page 65

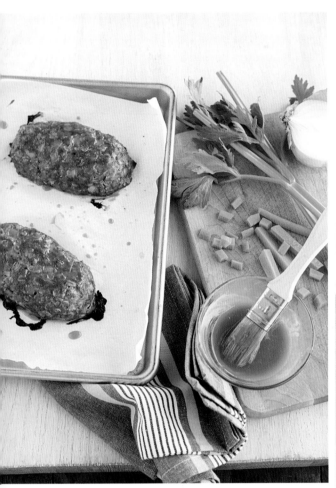

Turkey Mini Meat Loaf with
Dijon Glaze, page 124

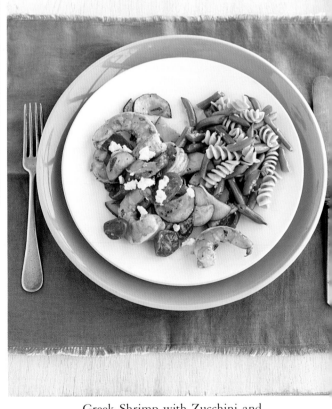

Greek Shrimp with Zucchini and
Grape Tomatoes, page 138

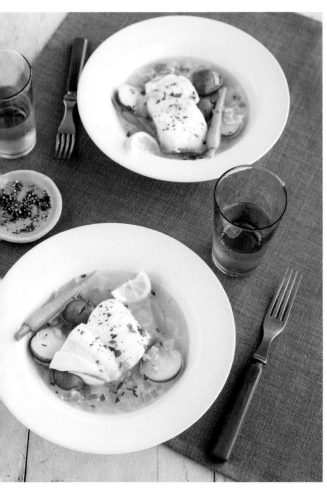

Halibut with Spring Vegetables, page 133

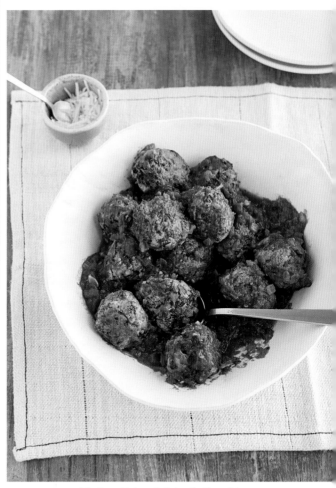

Turkey-Spinach Meatballs with
Tomato Sauce, page 120

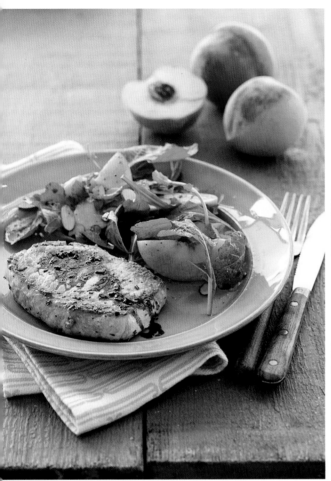

Rosemary Pork Chops with Balsamic Glaze, page 93;
Arugula, Peach, and Almond Salad, page 60

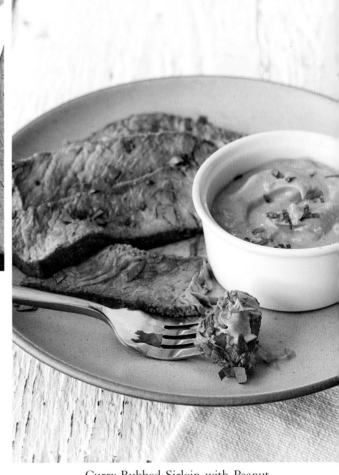

Curry-Rubbed Sirloin with Peanut
Dipping Sauce, page 77

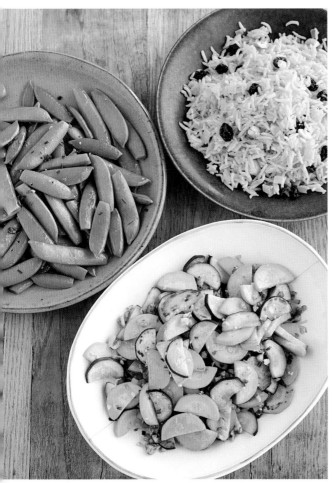

Sugar Snap Peas and Lemon Butter, page 178;
Indian Rice with Cashews, Raisins, and Spices, page 175;
Summer Squash and Walnut Sauté, page 179

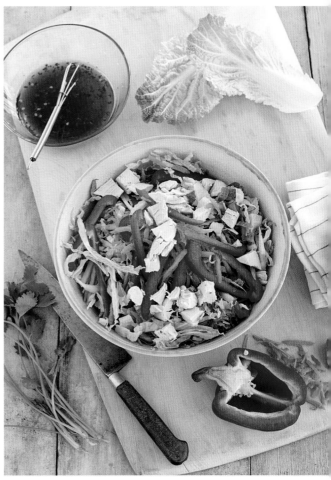

Chinese Chicken Salad, page 46

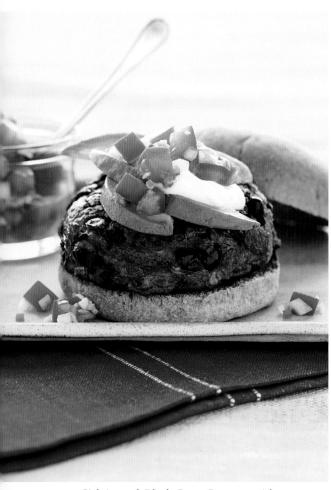

Sirloin and Black Bean Burgers with
Fresh Tomato Salsa, page 85

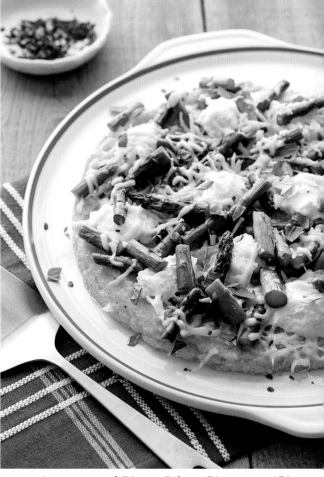

Asparagus and Ricotta Polenta Pizza, page 156

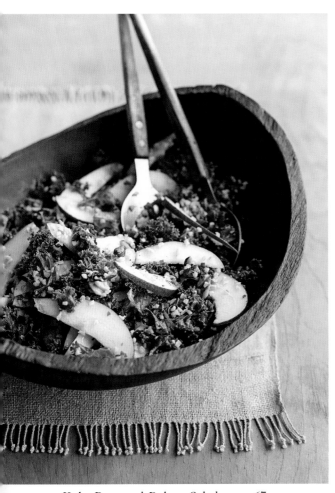

Kale, Pear, and Bulgur Salad, page 67

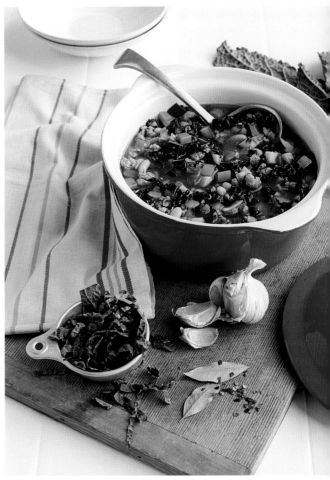

Sausage Minestrone with Kale
and Beans, page 32

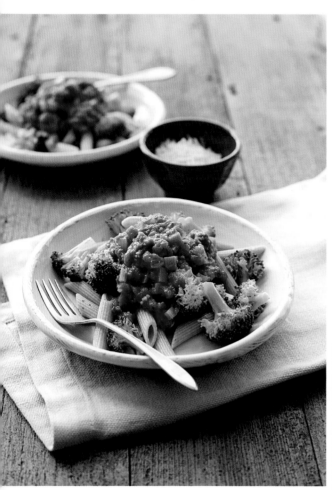

Beef Ragù with Broccoli Ziti, page 89

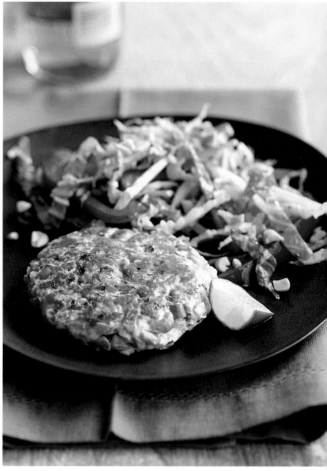

Salmon and Edamame Cakes, page 135;
Asian Slaw with Ginger Dressing, page 63

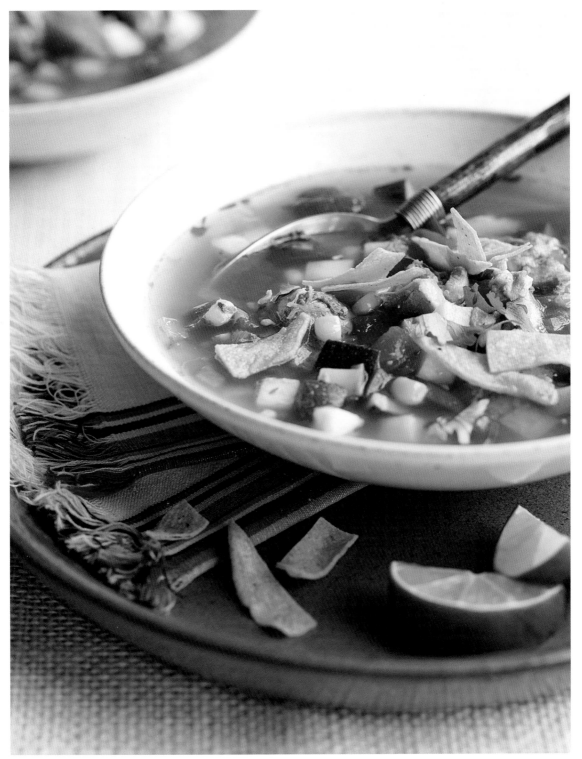

Mexican Chicken Tortilla Soup, page 28

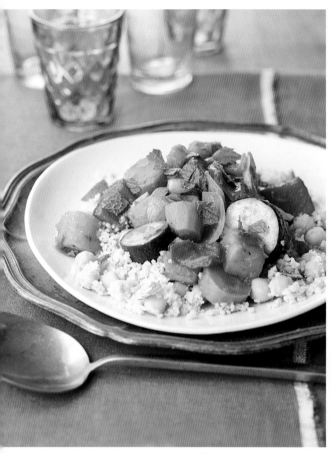

Moroccan Vegetables on
Garbanzo Couscous, page 151

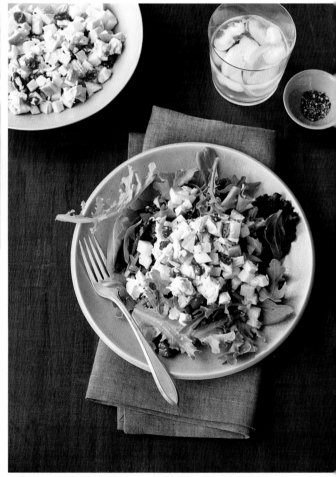

Autumn Turkey Salad with Apples
and Dried Cranberries, page 51

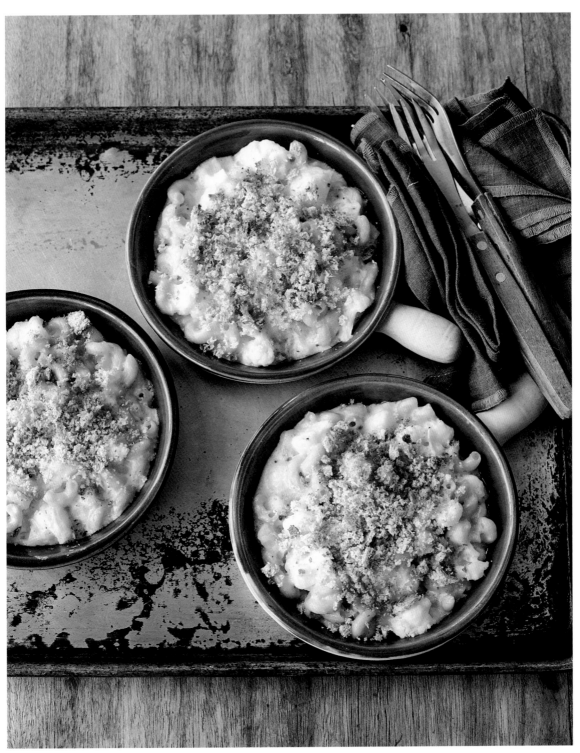

Cauliflower Macaroni and Cheese, page 145

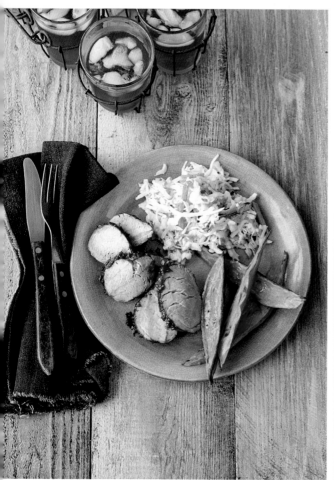

Pork Tenderloin with Easy BBQ Sauce, page 96;
Apple Coleslaw with Buttermilk Dressing, page 62;
Sweet Potato Steak Fries, page 181

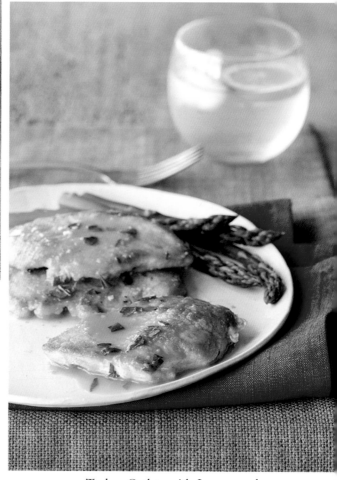

Turkey Cutlets with Lemon and
Basil Sauce, page 116

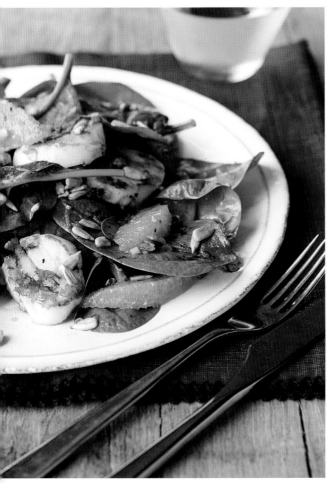

Warm Spinach Salad with Scallops and
Oranges, page 53

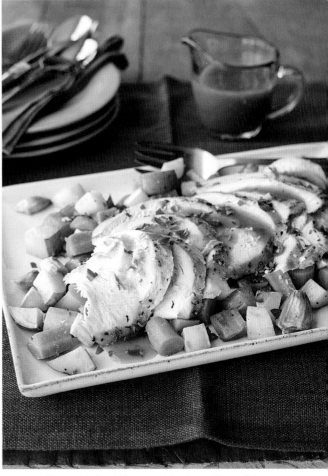

Roast Turkey Breast with Root Vegetables,
Lemon, and Garlic Cloves, page 114

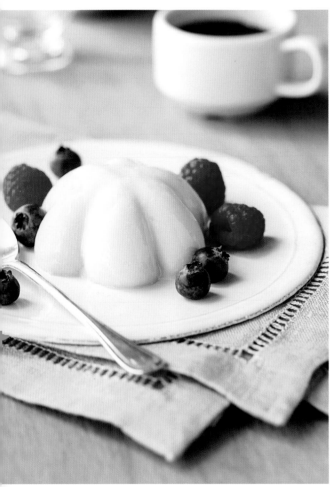

Buttermilk *Panna Cotta* with
Fresh Berries, page 187

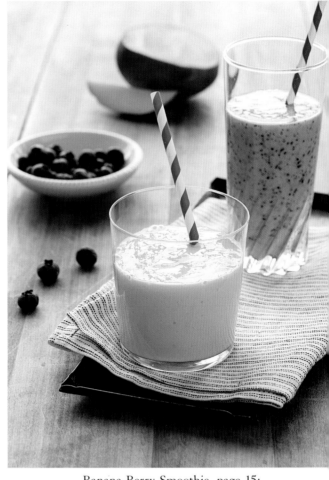

Banana-Berry Smoothie, page 15;
Mango Lassi, page 18

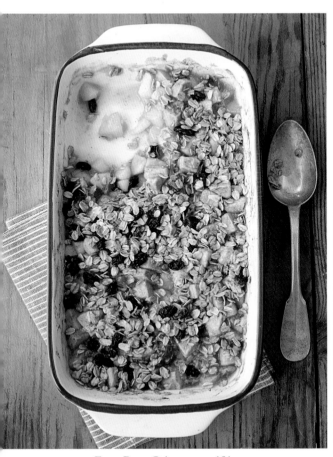

Easy Pear Crisp, page 191

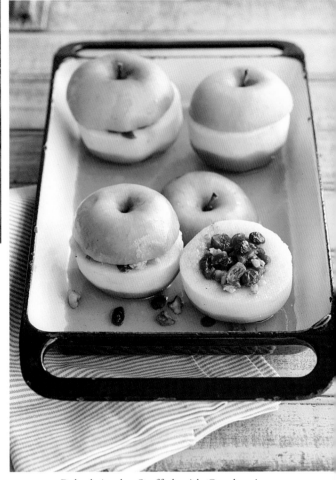

Baked Apples Stuffed with Cranberries
and Walnuts, page 185

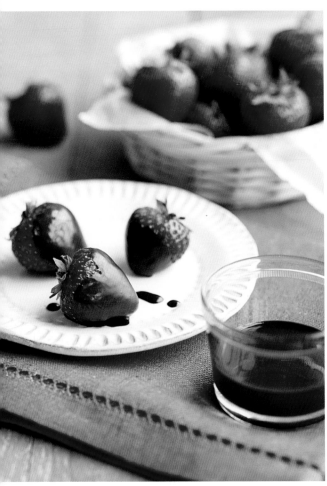

Fresh Strawberries with Chocolate Dip, page 193

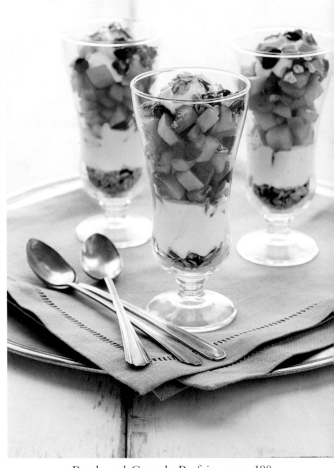

Peach and Granola Parfaits, page 190

Beef Ragù with Broccoli Ziti

There are few aromas more satisfying than ragù simmering on a stove, filling the kitchen with the appetizing scents of tomatoes, herbs, and garlic. This is pasta and sauce—the DASH way. Use ground sirloin in the sauce, and stretch the pasta with lots of vegetables. (You could also use the Green Beans and Fusilli on page 163.)   MAKES 6 SERVINGS

1 tablespoon olive oil

8 ounces ground sirloin

1 medium yellow onion, chopped

1 medium carrot, cut into ¼-inch dice

1 medium celery rib, cut into ¼-inch dice

2 cloves garlic, minced

1 (28-ounce) can no-salt-added crushed tomatoes

2 teaspoons Italian Seasoning (page xiv)

¼ teaspoon crushed hot red pepper

Broccoli Ziti (page 162)

6 tablespoons freshly grated Parmesan cheese (optional)

Heat the oil in a medium saucepan over medium-high heat. Add the beef and cook, stirring occasionally and breaking up the ground sirloin with the side of the spoon, until the meat loses its raw look, about 7 minutes. Stir in the onion, carrot, celery, and garlic. Reduce the heat to medium and cover. Cook, stirring occasionally, until the vegetables soften, about 5 minutes.

Stir in the tomatoes, Italian Seasoning, and hot pepper and bring to a boil. Reduce the heat to medium-low and simmer, stirring often, until the sauce has reduced slightly, about 45 minutes.

Divide the hot Broccoli Ziti among six deep bowls. Top each with an equal amount of sauce and sprinkle with 1 tablespoon Parmesan cheese, if using. Serve hot.

NUTRITIONAL ANALYSIS

(1 serving without cheese) 325 calories, 23 g protein, 38 g carbohydrates, 10 g fat, 6 g fiber, 47 mg cholesterol, 124 mg sodium, 1,087 mg potassium. Food groups: 3 ounces meat, 1 grain, 3 vegetables.

Tomato Time

You might be surprised to find that many tomato products—including tomatoes in juice, crushed tomatoes, and tomato paste—are available without additional salt; check the labels. In many cases, the small amount of sodium is occurring naturally from the tomatoes themselves. And tomatoes are loaded with potassium, and potassium-rich foods lower blood pressure by helping to excrete excess sodium.

Pork Chops in Mustard Sauce

All dinner entrées should be this easy and tasty. Remember that boneless pork chops should be cooked over medium heat and not overcooked. Keep that trick in mind and you will have a main course that you could serve to company. The herbs are optional, but a nice touch.
MAKES 4 SERVINGS (1½ CHOPS EACH)

Canola oil in a pump sprayer

6 (4-ounce) boneless pork loin chops, about ½ inch thick

½ teaspoon kosher salt

½ teaspoon freshly ground black pepper

2 teaspoons cornstarch

½ cup Homemade Chicken Broth (page 38) or canned low-sodium chicken broth

½ cup low-fat (1%) milk

1 tablespoon Dijon mustard

1 tablespoon unsalted butter

2 tablespoons minced shallots

2 teaspoons chopped fresh tarragon, rosemary, or chives

Spray a large nonstick skillet with oil and heat over medium heat. Season the pork with the salt and pepper and add to the skillet. Cook until the undersides are golden brown, about 3 minutes. Flip the pork and cook until the other sides are golden brown and the meat feels firm when pressed in the thickest part with a fingertip, about 3 minutes more. Transfer to a plate.

Meanwhile, in a small bowl whisk the cornstarch into the broth. Add the milk and mustard and whisk again; set aside.

Melt the butter in the skillet over medium heat. Add the shallots and cook, stirring often, until tender, about 2 minutes. Whisk the broth mixture again, pour into the skillet, and bring to a boil. Return the pork and any juices on the plate to the skillet and cook, turning occasionally, until the sauce thickens, about 1 minute. Transfer the pork to a deep platter and cut each chop in half. Pour the sauce over the pork chops and sprinkle with the tarragon. Serve hot.

NUTRITIONAL ANALYSIS

(1 serving) 207 calories, 25 g protein, 3 g carbohydrates, 10 g fat, 0 g fiber, 73 mg cholesterol, 323 mg sodium, 418 mg potassium. Food groups: 3½ ounces lean meat.

Pork Chops with Sweet-and-Sour Cabbage

I love sweet-and-sour red cabbage, especially when simmered with pork. It takes at least an hour of simmering to become tender and marry the flavors, so don't skimp on the time. This recipe makes a generous amount of cabbage, so you might have leftovers to serve at another meal.

MAKES 4 SERVINGS

Red Cabbage

1 slice reduced-sodium bacon, coarsely chopped

1 teaspoon canola oil

1 medium yellow onion, chopped

1 small red cabbage (1¼ pounds), cored and thinly sliced

¼ cup cider vinegar

2 Granny Smith apples, cored and cut into ½-inch dice

¼ cup water

3 tablespoons grade B maple syrup (see "Maple Syrup," page 92)

¼ teaspoon kosher salt

¼ teaspoon freshly ground black pepper

Pork Chops

Canola oil in a pump sprayer

4 (4-ounce) boneless center-cut pork chops, excess fat trimmed

¼ teaspoon kosher salt

¼ teaspoon freshly ground black pepper

To prepare the red cabbage: In a medium saucepan over medium heat, cook the bacon in the oil, stirring occasionally, until the bacon is crisp and brown, about 5 minutes. Add the onion and cook, stirring occasionally, until golden, about 5 minutes. In three or four additions, stir in the cabbage, sprinkling each addition with a tablespoon or so of the vinegar. Stir in the apples, water, maple syrup, salt, and pepper. Reduce the heat to medium-low and cover tightly. Cook, stirring occasionally, until the cabbage is very tender, about 1 hour. If the liquid cooks away, add a couple of tablespoons of water.

To prepare the pork: Spray a large nonstick skillet with oil and heat over medium heat. Season the pork with the salt and pepper and add to the skillet. Cook until the undersides are golden brown, about 3 minutes. Flip the pork and cook until the other sides are golden brown and the meat feels firm when pressed in the thickest part with a fingertip, about 3 minutes more. Transfer to a plate and tent with foil to keep warm.

Increase the heat under the skillet to high. Add the red cabbage mixture and any liquid to the skillet and cook, scraping up the browned bits in the skillet with a wooden spoon. Cook until the juices are thickened, about 3 minutes. Return the pork and any juices on the plate to the skillet. Serve hot.

NUTRITIONAL ANALYSIS

(1 serving) 356 calories, 29 g protein, 39 g carbohydrates, 10 g fat, 6 g fiber, 66 mg cholesterol, 377 mg sodium, 1,062 mg potassium.
Food groups: 3½ ounces meat, 2 vegetables, 1 fat, ½ fruit, 1 sugar.

Maple Syrup

Maple syrup is even more American than apple pie and was a sweetener on these shores long before sugar arrived. For the strongest maple flavor, buy grade B syrup (or "dark," its Canadian equivalent). This has a richer, deeper taste than grade A syrup (or Canadian no. 1 or no. 2), which should be reserved for topping pancakes and the like. The grades are not an indication of quality; they refer only to the syrup's depth of color and flavor. Grade B syrup is easy to find at natural food markets and many wholesale clubs.

Rosemary Pork Chops with Balsamic Glaze

Cooking with fresh herbs is one of the best ways to improve your everyday meals. There are many times when dried herbs will do, but this dish relies on just a few ingredients, so the bracing flavor of fresh rosemary is key. To keep the lean chops moist, cook them with medium heat so they brown at a steady pace without burning. MAKES 4 SERVINGS

Olive oil in a pump sprayer

4 (4-ounce) boneless pork loin chops, about ½ inch thick

1 tablespoon finely chopped fresh rosemary

½ teaspoon kosher salt

½ teaspoon freshly ground black pepper

¼ cup balsamic vinegar

Spray a large nonstick skillet with oil and heat over medium heat. Season the pork with the rosemary, salt, and pepper. Add to the skillet and cook until the undersides are golden brown, about 3 minutes. Flip the pork and cook, adjusting the heat as needed so the pork cooks steadily without burning, until the other sides are browned and the pork feels firm when pressed in the center with a fingertip, about 3 minutes more. Transfer each chop to a dinner plate.

Off heat, add the vinegar to the skillet. (Do not inhale the fumes, as they are strong.) Using a wooden spoon, scrape up the browned bits in the bottom of the skillet. The residual heat of the skillet should be enough to evaporate the vinegar to about 2 tablespoons. If necessary, return the skillet to medium heat to reduce the vinegar slightly. Drizzle the glaze over each chop and serve hot.

NUTRITIONAL ANALYSIS
(1 serving) 178 calories, 24 g protein, 3 g carbohydrates, 6 g fat, 0 g fiber, 67 mg cholesterol, 579 mg sodium, 376 mg potassium. Food groups: 3 ounces meat.

Cooking Pork

For decades, the USDA insisted that pork be cooked to 160°F for safe consumption, a temperature that most professional cooks believed caused overcooking and tough, dry meat. Recently, the recommended internal temperature for doneness has been lowered to 145°F, with a waiting period of 3 minutes before serving so the residual heat can raise the temperature a few more degrees. This yields pork that is juicy and tender, with a slightly pink cast to the meat.

Pork Chops with White Beans

A perfect warming rustic dish for an autumn evening; just serve a green salad on the side to make a substantial meal. This recipe is very high in soluble fiber, which is especially beneficial for helping to lower cholesterol.　　MAKES 4 SERVINGS

3 teaspoons olive oil

4 (4-ounce) boneless pork loin chops, about ½ inch thick

½ teaspoon kosher salt

½ teaspoon freshly ground black pepper

1 medium yellow onion, chopped

1 medium carrot, cut into ½-inch dice

1 medium celery rib, cut into ½-inch dice

2 cloves garlic, minced

½ cup Homemade Chicken Broth (page 38) or canned low-sodium chicken broth

1 (15-ounce) can no-salt-added cannellini beans, drained and rinsed

2 ripe plum (Roma) tomatoes, seeded and cut into ½-inch dice

½ teaspoon herbes de Provence, Italian Seasoning (page xiv), or dried rosemary

Chopped fresh parsley, for serving

Heat 1 teaspoon of the oil in a large nonstick skillet over medium heat. Season the pork with the salt and pepper. Add to the skillet and cook until the undersides are golden brown, about 3 minutes. Flip the chops and cook until the other sides are browned, about 3 minutes more. Transfer to a plate.

Heat the remaining 2 teaspoons oil in the skillet. Add the onion, carrot, celery, and garlic and cover. Cook, stirring occasionally, until the vegetables soften, about 5 minutes. Add the broth and bring to a simmer, stirring up the browned bits in the skillet with a wooden spoon. Stir in the beans, tomatoes, and herbes de Provence. Cover and simmer to blend the flavors, about 15 minutes.

Return the pork and any juices on the plate to the skillet. Simmer, uncovered, until the pork feels firm when pressed in the center with a fingertip, about 3 minutes.

Divide the bean mixture evenly among four large soup bowls and top each with a pork chop. Sprinkle with the parsley and serve.

NUTRITIONAL ANALYSIS
(1 serving) 458 calories, 33 g protein, 34 g carbohydrates, 21 g fat, 8 g fiber, 78 mg cholesterol, 357 mg sodium, 1,229 mg potassium. Food groups: 3 ounces meat, 2 beans, 1 vegetable, 2 fats.

NOTE: Many pork products that look natural are actually injected with salty liquid to help keep them moist during cooking. (The pork can still be labeled "all natural" because sodium is not chemically produced.) Look carefully at meat labels to be sure that you aren't buying pork that has been salted, or if you do buy these meats, include the sodium in your daily intake total.

Pork Tenderloin with Easy BBQ Sauce

With this simple recipe, you can enjoy the down-home flavor of barbecue without an overload of fat and calories. The tenderloin is browned first on the stove to develop flavor, then finished in the oven with a tangy glaze. (Be sure your skillet has an ovenproof handle.) If you really like spicy food, substitute a minced chipotle chili for the chili powder and liquid smoke. Serve this with Sweet Potato Steak Fries and Apple Coleslaw with Buttermilk Dressing (pages 181 and 62) for a country-style feast.   MAKES 6 SERVINGS

1½ pounds pork tenderloin, sinew and excess fat trimmed

1 teaspoon kosher salt

½ teaspoon freshly ground black pepper

1 tablespoon canola oil

2 tablespoons all-fruit peach spread

2 tablespoons no-salt-added tomato ketchup

1 tablespoon cider vinegar

1 teaspoon chili powder

½ teaspoon hickory liquid smoke flavoring (optional)

Preheat the oven to 350°F.

Season the pork with salt and pepper. Fold the thin ends of the tenderloin and tie them down with kitchen twine so the meat is evenly thick. Heat the oil in a large nonstick skillet with an ovenproof handle over medium heat. Add the tenderloin and cook, turning occasionally, until browned on all sides, about 5 minutes.

In a small bowl, mix the peach spread, ketchup, vinegar, chili powder, and liquid smoke (if using). Spread over the tenderloin. Transfer the skillet with the tenderloin to the oven and bake until an instant-read thermometer inserted in the center of the tenderloin reads 145°F, 12 to 15 minutes. Transfer the pork to a carving board and let stand for 5 minutes.

Remove the strings and cut the tenderloin crosswise into ½-inch-thick slices. Arrange on dinner plates and pour any carving juices on top. Serve hot.

NUTRITIONAL ANALYSIS
(1 serving: 4 ounces) 196 calories, 29 g protein, 6 g carbohydrates, 6 g fat, 0 g fiber, 88 mg cholesterol, 475 mg sodium, 579 mg potassium. Food groups: 4 ounces meat.

Grilled Pork and Vegetable Souvlaki with Oregano-Lemon Marinade

Souvlaki is the Greek version of shish kebab, and it is often made with lean pork. The marinade uses pureed onions and garlic to create a mixture that clings to the meat and delivers lots of flavor with every bite. You can grill the souvlaki on an outdoor grill over direct medium heat, if you wish. Chopped Greek Salad (page 65) will round out the meal. MAKES 6 SERVINGS

Marinade

½ cup coarsely chopped yellow onion

2 tablespoons fresh lemon juice

2 tablespoons olive oil, preferably extra-virgin

2 teaspoons dried oregano

2 garlic cloves, crushed under a knife and peeled

¼ teaspoon kosher salt

¼ teaspoon freshly ground black pepper

Souvlaki

1½ pounds center-cut pork loin, trimmed, and cut into eighteen 1½-inch pieces

1 medium red onion, peeled and cut into twelve 1½-inch pieces

1 large zucchini, trimmed, cut lengthwise and then crosswise into 12 pieces

Olive oil in a pump sprayer

Lemon wedges, for serving

To make the marinade: Puree the onion, lemon juice, oil, oregano, garlic, salt, and pepper together in a blender. Pour into a large zippered plastic bag.

To make the souvlaki: Add the pork to the bag and toss to coat with the marinade. Close the bag and refrigerate for at least 2 hours and up to 8 hours.

Position the broiler rack about 4 inches from the source of heat and preheat the broiler.

Have ready six metal kebab skewers. Remove the pork from the marinade, letting the marinade cling to the meat. Thread 3 pork pieces, 2 red onion pieces, and 2 zucchini pieces on each of six metal skewers, alternating the ingredients without packing them closely together. Spray the vegetables with oil.

Spray the broiler rack lightly with oil. Broil the souvlaki, turning occasionally, until the pork is lightly browned and is only barely pink when pierced with the tip of a small, sharp knife, 8 to 10 minutes. Remove from the broiler and let stand for 3 minutes. Serve hot with lemon wedges.

NUTRITIONAL ANALYSIS

(1 serving) 208 calories, 26 g protein, 8 g carbohydrates, 8 g fat, 2 g fiber, 73 mg cholesterol, 116 mg sodium, 697 mg potassium. Food groups: 3 ounces meat, 1 vegetable.

Kebab Skewers

Inexpensive metal kebab skewers are available at every supermarket. They are much easier to use than disposable bamboo skewers, which must be soaked before using and seem to burn under the broiler's heat no matter how long they are soaked. If you must use bamboo skewers, wrap the exposed ends of the skewers with aluminum foil to discourage scorching.

Pomegranate-Marinated Leg of Lamb

This lamb has an unusual marinade created from bottled pomegranate juice and other Mediterranean flavors. Because the marinade won't penetrate more than an eighth of an inch into the meat no matter how long it is soaked, an hour is sufficient. Cook it outside on the grill over direct medium heat when the weather cooperates. MAKES 6 SERVINGS

Marinade

½ cup bottled pomegranate juice

½ cup hearty red wine, such as Shiraz

1 teaspoon ground cumin

1 teaspoon dried oregano

½ teaspoon crushed hot red pepper

3 cloves garlic, minced

Lamb

1¾ pounds boneless leg of lamb, butterflied and surface fat trimmed

½ teaspoon kosher salt

Olive oil in a pump sprayer

To make the marinade: In a medium bowl, whisk together the pomegranate juice, wine, cumin, oregano, hot pepper, and garlic. Transfer to a large zippered plastic bag.

To prepare the lamb: Add the lamb to the bag, press out the air, and close the bag. Refrigerate, turning occasionally, for at least 1 hour and no longer than 8 hours.

Position a broiler rack about 8 inches from the source of heat and preheat the broiler.

Remove the lamb from the marinade, letting the excess marinade drip off. Blot with paper towels, but do not dry completely. Season with the salt. Spray the broiler rack with oil. Place the lamb on the rack and broil, turning occasionally, until browned and an instant-read thermometer inserted in the thickest part of the lamb reads 130°F for medium-rare, about 20 minutes. Transfer to a carving board and let stand for 5 minutes.

Cut the lamb across the grain into thin slices. Transfer to a platter and pour the carving juices on top. Serve hot.

NUTRITIONAL ANALYSIS
(1 serving) 273 calories, 31 g protein, 0 g carbohydrates, 15 g fat, 0 g fiber, 91 mg cholesterol, 219 mg sodium, 438 mg potassium. Food groups: 4 ounces meat.

Poultry

Lean poultry cuts (boneless, skinless chicken breast, turkey cutlets, and ground turkey) seem to be mainstays in every diet, and they certainly have their places. But without careful cooking, they can end up unappealingly dry and flavorless. My goal here is to show you how to cook the poultry correctly so you can truly enjoy it. (The main culprit is overcooking.)

As with red meat, I think sautéing in a nonstick skillet and then topping the chicken with a wonderful sauce loaded with vegetables is the best way to go. Here are a number of satisfying poultry recipes that are bound to become family favorites.

———————

Basic Roast Chicken Breast 101

For the tastiest chicken breast (and not just for dinner, but to have for sandwiches and salads), roast it intact and remove the skin and bone before eating. Many cooks season the skin before cooking, which is a mistake, because if you discard the skin, the seasoning goes with it. The solution is to pull back the skin, season the flesh, and replace the skin. This trick will save you from serving dried-out chicken breast ever again. A quick pan sauce finishes the dish. (It is interesting to note the relatively small amount of fat provided by the butter.) If you wish, rub ¼ teaspoon of your favorite dried herb (or ½ teaspoon of a finely chopped fresh herb) on the flesh of each breast, too. Rosemary or tarragon is especially good with roast chicken.

MAKES 4 SERVINGS

2 (10-ounce) chicken breast halves, with skin and bone

½ teaspoon kosher salt

¼ teaspoon freshly ground black pepper

Olive oil in a pump sprayer

1 tablespoon minced shallot

⅔ cup Homemade Chicken Broth (page 38) or canned low-sodium chicken broth; or ½ cup chicken broth plus 2 tablespoons dry vermouth or dry white wine

1 tablespoon cold unsalted butter (optional)

Preheat the oven to 400°F.

Work with one breast half at a time: Starting at the rib cage, use a small, sharp knife to cut away the skin from the flesh and pull back the skin, keeping it attached at the wide side of the chicken half. Season the exposed flesh with the salt and pepper. Replace the skin, covering the flesh.

Arrange the chicken skin side up in a small roasting pan (a metal 9 × 13-inch baking dish works well) and spray with the oil. Roast until an instant-read thermometer inserted in the thickest part of the chicken registers 165°F, 35 to 40 minutes. Transfer the chicken to a carving board and let stand for 5 minutes. (If you are preparing the chicken specifically for salads and sandwiches, let cool completely. You may choose to skip the next step.)

Pour off all but 1 teaspoon of the fat from the pan. Add the shallot to the pan and cook over medium heat, stirring often, until the shallot softens, about 1 minute. Add the broth and bring to a boil over high heat, scraping up the browned bits in the pan with a wooden spoon. Boil until the broth has reduced by one-third, about 2 minutes. Remove from the heat. If you wish to thicken the sauce slightly, add the butter to the pan sauce and whisk until the butter melts.

Carve the meat from the chicken, discarding the skin and bones. Transfer to dinner plates and drizzle equal amounts of the sauce over each serving. Serve hot.

NUTRITIONAL ANALYSIS

(1 serving, without butter) 138 calories, 21 g protein, 1 g carbohydrates, 5 g fat, 0 g fiber, 62 mg cholesterol, 370 mg sodium, 400 mg potassium. Food groups: 3 ounces lean meat.

(1 serving, with butter) 165 calories, 21 g protein, 1 g carbohydrates, 8 g fat (3 g saturated fat), 69 mg cholesterol, 370 mg sodium, 400 mg potassium. Food groups: 3 ounces lean meat.

(1 serving, with wine and butter in the sauce) 168 calories, 21 g protein, 1 g carbohydrates, 8 g fat (3 g saturated fat), 69 mg cholesterol, 367 mg sodium, 400 mg potassium. Food groups: 3 ounces lean meat.

Classic Poached Chicken

If you are cooking chicken specifically for salad, try this stovetop method, which uses gentle heat to keep the meat moist and flavorful. You'll have a bonus of homemade chicken broth, too.

MAKES ABOUT 2½ CUPS DICED CHICKEN MEAT

2 (10-ounce) chicken breast halves, with skin and bones

1 small onion, thinly sliced

2 sprigs of fresh parsley (optional)

Pinch of dried thyme

A few black peppercorns

½ bay leaf

In a medium saucepan, place the chicken and onion and add enough water to cover by 1 inch (about 1 quart). Bring to a simmer over high heat, skimming off any foam that rises to the surface.

Add the parsley (if using) and the thyme, peppercorns, and bay leaf. Reduce the heat to medium-low and simmer for 15 minutes. The chicken will not be completely cooked.

Remove from the heat and cover tightly. Let stand until the chicken is opaque when pierced in the thickest part with the tip of a knife, about 20 minutes. Transfer the chicken to a cutting board and let cool until easy to handle.

Pull off the skin and bones. (If you want to make chicken broth, return the skin and bones to the saucepan. Simmer over low heat until the liquid is reduced to about 2 cups, about 1 hour. Strain into a heatproof bowl and cool. Refrigerate in an airtight container for up to 3 days or freeze for up to 2 months.) Cover and refrigerate the meat for up to 2 days.

NUTRITIONAL ANALYSIS
(1 serving: 4 ounces or ¾ cup of ½-inch diced cooked chicken) 194 calories, 33 g protein, 4 g carbohydrates, 4 g fat, 1 g fiber, 100 mg cholesterol, 183 mg sodium, 641 mg potassium. Food groups: 4 ounces meat.

Chicken Mediterranean with Artichokes and Rosemary

The bright flavors of Italian cuisine make this weeknight dish sing. If you feel like splurging, top each piece of chicken with 2 tablespoons of shredded reduced-fat mozzarella cheese during the last 2 minutes of cooking. **MAKES 4 SERVINGS**

1 tablespoon olive oil, plus more in a pump sprayer

2 (12-ounce) boneless, skinless chicken breasts, pounded to even thickness, each cut in half crosswise to make 4 serving pieces (see note)

1 teaspoon kosher salt

¼ teaspoon freshly ground black pepper

½ small yellow onion, chopped

½ large red bell pepper, seeded and cut into ½-inch dice

1 clove garlic, minced

1 (14.5-ounce) no-salt-added diced tomatoes in juice, drained

1 (9-ounce) box thawed frozen artichoke hearts, coarsely chopped

2 teaspoons cornstarch

1 cup Homemade Chicken Broth (page 38) or canned low-sodium chicken broth

2 teaspoons chopped fresh rosemary or sage, or 1 teaspoon dried rosemary or sage

¼ teaspoon crushed hot red pepper

Spray a large nonstick skillet with oil and heat over medium heat. Season the chicken with the salt and pepper. Add the chicken to the skillet and cook, turning halfway through cooking, until golden brown on both sides, about 6 minutes. Transfer to a plate.

Heat the 1 tablespoon oil in the skillet over medium heat. Add the onion, bell pepper, and garlic and cook, stirring occasionally, until softened, about 5 minutes. Stir in the tomatoes and artichokes. In a small bowl, dissolve the cornstarch in the broth. Stir into the skillet mixture, along with the rosemary and hot pepper. Return the chicken to the skillet and bring the liquid to a simmer. Reduce the heat to medium-low and cover the skillet with the lid ajar. Cook, stirring occasionally, until the juices are lightly thickened and the chicken is opaque when pierced in the thickest part with the tip of a knife, about 6 minutes. Serve hot.

NUTRITIONAL ANALYSIS

(1 serving) 300 calories, 40 g protein, 15 g carbohydrates, 9 g fat, 5 g fiber, 109 mg cholesterol, 534 mg sodium, 914 mg potassium. Food groups: 5 ounces meat, ½ fat, 1 vegetable.

NOTE: As an indication of how the American serving size has grown out of proportion, check the average weight of the boneless, skinless chicken breast halves at your local market. When I was testing these recipes, the chicken breast halves averaged 10 to 12 ounces, especially when purchased in the "value" or "family" packs. I cut these portions in half before cooking to make more reasonably sized servings. If you have children in your family or others with smaller appetites, you may be able to stretch this meal to serve six people.

Pounding Chicken Breasts

Boneless, skinless chicken breast halves are ubiquitous in the American diet. But their irregular shape (uneven thickness, plump in the middle, tapering to thinner ends) can cause problems with cooking. Taking a few seconds to pound the meat into an evenly thick shape resolves the issue. Place the chicken breast half on a cutting board and top with a plastic storage bag. Using the flat side of a meat mallet (or a rolling pin), pound the chicken, concentrating on the plump central area, so it is ¾ to 1 inch thick. Don't pummel the chicken so it falls apart. Just a few well-placed, strong blows should do the trick.

Chinese Chicken with Bok Choy and Garlic

Like its cousins in the cruciferous vegetable family, bok choy is a nutrition powerhouse packed with antioxidants. Sometimes I will add sliced shiitake mushroom caps to the bok choy, but this is the basic recipe with chicken for added protein. (It is also delicious with sliced boneless pork loin.) **MAKES 4 SERVINGS**

Sauce

¾ cup Homemade Chicken Broth (page 38) or canned low-sodium chicken broth

2 tablespoons rice vinegar

1 tablespoon reduced-sodium soy sauce

1 teaspoon amber agave nectar or sugar

½ teaspoon crushed hot red pepper

2 teaspoons cornstarch

Chicken

4 teaspoons canola oil

1 pound boneless, skinless chicken breast halves, cut across the grain into ¼-inch-thick slices

4 cloves garlic, minced

2 tablespoons peeled and minced fresh ginger

1 large head bok choy (1½ pounds), cut crosswise into ½-inch-thick pieces, well washed, but not dried

3 scallions, white and green parts, cut into 1-inch lengths

To make the sauce: In a small bowl, mix the broth, vinegar, soy sauce, agave, and hot pepper. Sprinkle in the cornstarch and stir to dissolve. Set the sauce mixture aside.

To prepare the chicken: Heat 2 teaspoons of the oil in a large wok or nonstick skillet over medium-high heat. Add the chicken and cook, stirring occasionally, until lightly browned, about 2 minutes. Transfer to a plate.

Heat the remaining 2 teaspoons oil in the skillet. Add the garlic and ginger and stir until fragrant, about 30 seconds. Add the bok choy and scallions and cook, stirring often, until the bok choy is crisp-tender, about 3 minutes. Return the chicken and any juices on the plate to the skillet. Cook, stirring often, until the chicken is opaque throughout, about 1 minute. Stir in the sauce mixture and cook, stirring often, until boiling and lightly thickened. Serve hot.

NUTRITIONAL ANALYSIS
(1 serving) 225 calories, 28 g protein, 10 g carbohydrates, 8 g fat, 2 g fiber, 72 mg cholesterol, 409 mg sodium, 951 mg potassium. Food groups: 3½ ounces meat, 2 vegetables.

Chicken with Mushroom Cacciatore Sauce

Cacciatore means "hunter" in Italian, and assuming that a hunter would forage in the woods, mushrooms are often featured in cacciatore sauce. Cremini (baby bella) mushrooms are more flavorful than white mushrooms, so use them if you can. People with smaller appetites will have leftovers for another meal.   MAKES 4 SERVINGS

1 tablespoon olive oil, plus more in a pump sprayer

2 (12-ounce) boneless, skinless chicken breast halves, pounded to even thickness, each cut in half crosswise to make 4 serving pieces

½ teaspoon kosher salt

¼ teaspoon freshly ground black pepper

1 medium yellow onion, chopped

½ medium green bell pepper, cored and cut into ½-inch dice

1 clove garlic, minced

1 (14.5-ounce) can no-salt-added diced tomatoes with juice, undrained

¼ cup hearty red wine, dry vermouth, or water

1 teaspoon Italian herb seasoning or dried oregano

Spray a large nonstick skillet with oil and heat over medium heat. Season the chicken with the salt and pepper, add to the skillet, and cook, turning halfway through cooking, until golden brown on both sides, about 6 minutes. Transfer to a plate.

Heat the 1 tablespoon oil in the skillet over medium heat. Add the onion, bell pepper, and garlic and cook, stirring occasionally, until softened, about 5 minutes. Stir in the tomatoes with their juice, the wine, and the herb seasoning. Bring to a simmer, scraping up the browned bits in the skillet with a wooden spoon. Reduce the heat to medium-low and simmer until the liquid is slightly reduced, about 5 minutes.

Return the chicken to the skillet and cover with the lid ajar. Simmer until the chicken is opaque when pierced in the thickest part with the tip of a sharp knife, 6 to 8 minutes. Serve hot.

NUTRITIONAL ANALYSIS
(1 serving) 281 calories, 38 g protein, 10 g carbohydrates, 8 g fat, 3 g fiber, 109 mg cholesterol, 733 mg sodium, 749 mg potassium. Food groups: 5½ ounces meat, 2 vegetables.

(For smaller appetites: 1 serving, with recipe divided into 6 servings) 188 calories, 25 g protein, 7 g carbohydrates, 1 g fat, 2 g fiber, 73 mg cholesterol, 489 mg sodium, 500 mg potassium. Food groups: 3½ ounces meat, 1 vegetable.

Mexican Chicken Breast with Tomatillo Salsa

Tomatillos, which are actually related to gooseberries and not tomatoes, are the main ingredient in the classic green Mexican salsa. It is surprisingly easy to make and good to have on hand to add a tart jolt of flavor to your food or to serve with baked tortilla strips as a dip. Here it dresses up sautéed chicken breast. Serve it with the Black Beans and Brown Rice on page 159 for a Mexican dinner at home.   MAKES 4 SERVINGS

Tomatillo Sauce

8 ounces tomatillos (preferably all the same size), husked

2 scallions, white and green parts, coarsely chopped

½ jalapeño, seeded and minced

1 tablespoon fresh lime juice

1 tablespoon coarsely chopped fresh cilantro

1 clove garlic, crushed under a knife and peeled

Pinch of kosher salt

Chicken

Olive oil in a pump sprayer

2 (10-ounce) boneless, skinless chicken breast halves, pounded to ¾-inch thickness and cut in half to make 4 portions

1 tablespoon Mexican Seasoning (page xiv)

Lime wedges, for serving

To make the sauce: Bring a medium saucepan of water to a boil over high heat. Add the tomatillos and reduce the heat to medium. Cook at a moderate boil just until they turn olive green, using a slotted spoon to transfer the tomatillos from the water to a bowl as they are ready, about 5 minutes. Do not overcook or the tomatillos will burst. Carefully drain the tomatillos.

In a food processor (or a blender with its lid ajar), puree the drained tomatillos, scallions, jalapeño, lime juice, cilantro, garlic, and salt. Set aside.

To prepare the chicken: Spray a large nonstick skillet with oil and heat over medium heat. Spray the chicken on both sides with the oil and sprinkle with the Mexican Seasoning. Add the chicken to the skillet and cook, turning halfway through cooking, until golden brown on both sides, about 6 minutes.

Pour in the tomatillo salsa and simmer until the chicken is opaque when pierced in the thickest part with the tip of a sharp knife, 6 to 8 minutes. Serve hot with the lime wedges.

NUTRITIONAL ANALYSIS
(1 serving) 190 calories, 31 g protein, 6 g carbohydrates, 4 g fat, 2 g fiber, 91 mg cholesterol, 208 mg sodium, 740 mg potassium. Food groups: 4½ ounces meat, 1 vegetable.

Chicken and Apple Curry

Chicken curry with a difference, this version is also loaded with fruit and vegetables. For a hotter curry, add ⅛ teaspoon cayenne with the curry powder. Spoon the curry over Basic Brown Rice (page 174), and sprinkle each serving with 2 tablespoons dark raisins, if you like.

MAKES 4 SERVINGS

2 teaspoons canola oil, plus more in a pump sprayer

2 (10-ounce) boneless, skinless chicken breast halves, trimmed, pounded to ¾-inch thickness, and cut into 4 equal serving portions

1 medium yellow onion, chopped

2 medium celery ribs, chopped

2 Granny Smith apples, peeled, cored, and cut into ½-inch dice

1 tablespoon curry powder

¾ cup light coconut milk

½ cup water

2 tablespoons fresh lime juice

½ cup sliced natural almonds, for serving

Spray a large nonstick skillet with oil and heat over medium-high heat. Add the chicken and cook, flipping halfway through cooking, until lightly browned on both sides, about 6 minutes. Transfer to a plate.

Heat the 2 teaspoons oil in the skillet over medium heat. Add the onion, celery, and apples and cook, stirring often, until the onion is tender, about 5 minutes. Sprinkle in the curry powder and stir well.

Stir in the coconut milk, water, and lime juice and bring to a simmer, stirring often. Add the chicken and cover. Reduce the heat to medium-low and simmer until the chicken is opaque when pierced in the center with the tip of a small, sharp knife, about 6 minutes.

Transfer the chicken to a deep serving platter. Increase the heat under the skillet to high and boil the sauce until lightly thickened, about 1 minute. Pour the sauce mixture over the chicken and sprinkle with the almonds. Serve hot.

NUTRITIONAL ANALYSIS
(1 serving) 444 calories, 35 g protein, 26 g carbohydrates, 24 g fat, 7 g fiber, 91 mg cholesterol, 192 mg sodium, 1,007 mg potassium. Food groups: 5 ounces meat, 1 fruit, ½ nuts.

(1 serving, with recipe divided into 6 servings) 296 calories, 23 g protein, 17 g carbohydrates, 16 g fat, 4 g fiber, 60 mg cholesterol, 128 mg sodium, 671 mg potassium. Food groups: 3 ounces meat, ½ fruit.

"Moo Shu" Chicken and Vegetable Wraps

Owing to their high sodium content, most Chinese condiments (such as soy sauce, oyster sauce, and hoisin sauce) should be used in moderation. In this variation on moo shu chicken, I've created my own hoisin sauce and substituted the hard-to-find vegetables with broccoli slaw.   MAKES 6 SERVINGS

Sauce

⅓ cup Homemade Chicken Broth (page 38) or canned low-sodium chicken broth

1 tablespoon rice vinegar

1 tablespoon no-salt-added tomato ketchup

1 tablespoon reduced-sodium soy sauce

1 teaspoon Asian sesame oil

2 teaspoons cornstarch

Chicken

4 teaspoons canola oil

1 (8-ounce) boneless, skinless chicken breast half, cut across the grain into ¼-inch-thick bite-sized pieces

10 ounces shiitake mushroom caps, sliced

1 (12-ounce) package broccoli slaw

3 scallions, white and green parts, cut into 1-inch lengths

1 (8-ounce) can sliced water chestnuts, drained and rinsed

1 tablespoon peeled and minced fresh ginger

2 cloves garlic, minced

Wraps

12 Boston or Bibb lettuce leaves

To make the sauce: In a small bowl, whisk together the broth, vinegar, ketchup, soy sauce, sesame oil, and cornstarch.

To prepare the chicken: Heat 2 teaspoons of the oil in a large nonstick skillet over medium-high heat. Add the chicken and cook, stirring occasionally, until it turns opaque throughout, about 4 minutes. Transfer to a plate.

Heat the remaining 2 teaspoons oil in the skillet over medium-high heat. Add the mushrooms and cook, stirring occasionally, until softened, about 5 minutes. Add the broccoli slaw, scallions, and water chestnuts and cook, stirring often, until the slaw is hot and wilted, about 3 minutes. Add the ginger and garlic and cook until fragrant, about 1 minute more. Stir the reserved chicken and sauce mixture and add to the skillet. Stir until the sauce is thickened and boiling, about 30 seconds.

To serve, transfer the chicken mixture to a serving bowl. Let each person spoon the chicken mixture onto a lettuce leaf, roll it up, and enjoy.

NUTRITIONAL ANALYSIS

(1 serving: 2 wraps) 144 calories, 11 g protein, 15 g carbohydrates, 5 g fat, 4 g fiber, 24 mg cholesterol, 168 mg sodium, 397 mg potassium. Food groups: 1½ ounces meat, 3 vegetables, 1 fat.

Roast Turkey Breast with Root Vegetables, Lemon, and Garlic Cloves

Roast a turkey breast half, and you will get a generous amount of meat with enough to reserve for salad at another meal. In fact, you may want to roast 2 breast halves in the same pan to ensure leftovers. Many supermarkets carry turkey breast halves weighing 2½ to 3 pounds, but if your butcher has only the large whole breast, ask to have it split in half lengthwise. Think this recipe calls for a lot of garlic? Don't worry. The roasting process creates a very soft, mellow flavor. If you like roasted garlic, eat the cloves; if not, discard them.

MAKES 6 SERVINGS

1 (2¾-pound) turkey breast half, with skin and bones

1 teaspoon herbes de Provence or Italian Seasoning (page xiv)

1 teaspoon kosher salt

¾ teaspoon freshly ground black pepper

2 pounds red-skinned potatoes, cut into 1-inch pieces

3 large carrots, cut into 1-inch pieces

2 medium parsnips, peeled and cut into 1-inch pieces

1 medium turnip, peeled and cut into 1-inch pieces

1 head garlic, separated into unpeeled cloves

1 tablespoon olive oil

Grated zest of 1 lemon

2 tablespoons fresh lemon juice

1 tablespoon cornstarch

1½ cups Homemade Chicken Broth (page 38) or canned low-sodium chicken broth

Chopped fresh parsley, for garnish

Preheat the oven to 350°F.

Using a small, sharp knife, make a narrow incision in the turkey breast to separate the skin from the rib bones. Slip your fingers under the skin to make a pocket. Season the flesh under the skin with the herbes de Provence, ½ teaspoon of the salt, and ½ teaspoon of the pepper.

In a large roasting pan, combine the potatoes, carrots, parsnips, turnip, and garlic. Drizzle with the oil and toss well. Spread in the pan and top with the turkey.

Roast until the turkey is golden brown and an instant-read thermometer inserted in the thickest part of the breast half registers 165°F, about 1½ hours. Transfer the turkey to a carving board and tent with aluminum foil.

Increase the oven temperature to 450°F. Continue cooking the vegetables in the roasting pan, stirring occasionally, until tender and lightly browned, about 10 minutes. Remove from the oven. Add the lemon zest and juice, the remaining ½ teaspoon salt, and the remaining ¼ teaspoon pepper and toss well. Transfer to a serving platter and tent with aluminum foil to keep warm.

Pour out and discard the fat in the pan. In a small bowl, sprinkle the cornstarch over the broth and stir until dissolved. Heat the roasting pan over medium-high heat until sizzling. Pour in the broth mixture and bring to a boil, scraping up the browned bits in the pan with a wooden spoon. Reduce the heat to low and simmer until lightly thickened, about 2 minutes. Pour the sauce into a gravy boat.

Discard the turkey skin. Carve the turkey meat from the bone across the grain in ½-inch-thick slices. Arrange the turkey over the vegetables and sprinkle with the parsley. Serve hot with the sauce.

NUTRITIONAL ANALYSIS
(1 serving) 355 calories, 40 g protein, 45 g carbohydrates, 2 g fat, 7 g fiber, 94 mg cholesterol, 495 mg sodium, 1,524 mg potassium. Food groups: 4 ounces meat, 3 starchy vegetables, 1 vegetable.

Turkey Cutlets with Lemon and Basil Sauce

Lean turkey breast is the perfect protein for a low-fat dinner. And fresh lemon juice and zest give this dish a lovely flavor. An important tip: Use medium heat and take care not to overcook the turkey or the cutlets will be tough and dry. The sauce is great with fresh basil (what isn't?), but you can substitute fresh parsley, tarragon, or rosemary. To remove the lemon zest, use a rasp-type zester—it makes the job fast and easy. MAKES 4 SERVINGS

1 pound turkey cutlets, cut into 8 serving pieces

½ teaspoon kosher salt

¼ teaspoon freshly ground black pepper

¼ cup whole-wheat flour

4 teaspoons olive oil

1 cup Homemade Chicken Broth (page 38) or canned low-sodium chicken broth

Grated zest of ½ lemon

3 tablespoons fresh lemon juice

2 tablespoons dry vermouth

1 tablespoon cold unsalted butter

2 tablespoons finely chopped fresh basil

Season the turkey with the salt and pepper. Spread the flour on a plate, and coat the turkey with the flour, shaking off the excess. Heat 2 teaspoons of the oil in a large nonstick skillet over medium heat. Add half of the turkey to the skillet and cook, flipping the turkey halfway through cooking, until lightly browned on both sides, about 4 minutes. Transfer to a plate. Repeat with the remaining 2 teaspoons oil and the turkey, and add to the turkey on the plate.

Combine the broth, lemon zest and juice, and vermouth in the skillet and bring to a boil over high heat. Cook until reduced by half, about 5 minutes. Return all of the turkey to the skillet and reduce the heat to medium. Cook, turning the turkey in the sauce, until the sauce is lightly thickened and the turkey is opaque when pierced in the center with the tip of a sharp knife, about 2 minutes. Transfer the turkey to a serving platter.

Remove the skillet from the heat. Whisk in the butter, then 1 tablespoon of the basil. Pour over the turkey, and sprinkle with the remaining 1 tablespoon basil. Serve hot.

NUTRITIONAL ANALYSIS
(1 serving) 208 calories, 29 g protein, 2 g carbohydrates, 8 g fat, 0 g fiber, 52 mg cholesterol, 365 mg sodium, 78 mg potassium. Food groups: 4 ounces very lean meat, 2 fats.

Dry Vermouth

There is a good reason many recipes have wine in them: Alcohol brings out the flavor of the other ingredients, while supplying its own taste. Alcohol is high in calories, which makes drinking it by the glass an indulgence, but it can be used in small amounts in cooking.

Dry white wine is a common cooking ingredient, but what do you do with the leftover wine before it goes bad if you aren't going to drink it? Dry vermouth, which is white wine infused with herbs and spices and fortified with brandy, is a great substitute. It will keep, tightly capped in its bottle, for a couple of months stored in the refrigerator. Don't store it at room temperature or its flavor will be compromised and its shelf life shortened.

Sloppy Toms

Sloppy Joes are a family favorite, but they can be made in a much more healthful manner with ground turkey, more vegetables than usual, less sugar, and reduced-sodium products. About half of the sodium and calories here comes from the bun. If you know you are going to serve this for dinner, watch your bread consumption during the day so you can have a whole bun at dinner. Or if you're seriously limiting starch, skip it.   MAKES 4 CUPS

1 tablespoon canola oil

1 medium yellow onion, chopped

2 large celery ribs, cut into ½-inch dice

1 large green bell pepper, cored and cut into ½-inch dice

1¼ pounds ground turkey

1 (8-ounce) can no-salt-added tomato sauce

½ cup no-salt-added tomato ketchup

1 tablespoon Worcestershire sauce

1 tablespoon balsamic vinegar

1 teaspoon kosher salt

½ teaspoon freshly ground black pepper

6 whole-wheat sandwich buns, toasted

Heat the oil in a large nonstick skillet over medium heat. Add the onion, celery, and bell pepper and sauté, stirring occasionally, until softened, about 5 minutes. Move the vegetables to one side of the skillet. Add the ground turkey to the cleared side of the skillet and cook, stirring occasionally and breaking up the meat with the side of a wooden spoon, until the turkey loses its raw look, about 6 minutes. Mix the turkey and vegetables.

Stir in the tomato sauce, ketchup, Worcestershire sauce, vinegar, salt, and pepper and bring to a simmer. Reduce the heat to medium-low and simmer, stirring often, until slightly thickened, about 10 minutes.

For each serving, spoon ⅔ cup of the turkey mixture onto half a bun on a plate, then cover with the top half of the bun. Serve hot.

NUTRITIONAL ANALYSIS

(1 serving, without bun) 222 calories, 18 g protein, 15 g carbo-hydrates, 12 g fat, 2 g fiber, 70 mg cholesterol, 389 mg sodium, 626 mg potassium. Food groups: 2½ ounces meat, ½ vegetable.

(1 serving, with bun) 382 calories, 24 g protein, 45 g carbohy-drates, 13 g fat, 7 g fiber, 70 mg cholesterol, 715 mg sodium, 767 mg potassium. Food groups: 2 whole grains, 2½ ounces meat, ½ vegetable.

NOTE: About half the sodium and calories comes from the bun. If you want to reduce them, have the Sloppy Toms without the bun and add extra vegetables. Did you know that bread is the number one source of sodium in the typical American diet?

Turkey-Spinach Meatballs with Tomato Sauce

This dish is satisfying enough to serve without pasta (although you could serve it with the Broccoli Ziti on page 162).

MAKES 6 SERVINGS

Turkey-Spinach Meatballs

1 (10-ounce) box frozen chopped spinach, thawed and squeezed to remove excess liquid

1 medium yellow onion, shredded on the large holes of a box grater

2 cloves garlic, minced

⅓ cup whole-wheat bread crumbs, made from day-old bread pulsed in the blender

2 large egg whites, or ¼ cup seasoned liquid egg substitute

1 teaspoon Italian Seasoning (page xiv) or dried oregano

1 teaspoon kosher salt

½ teaspoon freshly ground black pepper

1¼ pounds ground turkey

Olive oil in a pump sprayer

½ cup water

Tomato Sauce

1 tablespoon olive oil

1 medium yellow onion, chopped

2 cloves garlic, minced

1 (28-ounce) can no-salt-added crushed tomatoes

To make the meatballs: In a large bowl, mix the spinach, onion, garlic, bread crumbs, egg whites, Italian Seasoning, salt, and pepper. Add the ground turkey and combine thoroughly. Refrigerate for 15 to 30 minutes to firm the mixture and make it easier to handle.

Roll the turkey mixture into 18 meatballs. Spray a large nonstick skillet with oil and heat over medium heat. In batches, add the meatballs and cook, turning occasionally, until lightly browned, about 6 minutes. Transfer to a plate. Add the water to the skillet and bring to a boil, stirring up the browned bits in the pan with a wooden spoon. Remove from the heat.

To make the sauce: Heat the oil in a medium saucepan over medium heat. Add the onion and sauté, stirring occasionally, until golden and tender, about 5 minutes. Stir in the garlic and cook until fragrant, about 1 minute. Add the liquid from the skillet, the tomatoes, Italian Seasoning, and hot pepper; combine thoroughly and bring to a boil. Reduce the heat to medium-low and simmer, stirring occasionally, until lightly thickened, about 15 minutes. Bury the meatballs in the sauce and cook until the meatballs show no sign of pink when pierced to the center with the tip of a sharp knife, about 15 minutes more. Divide

2 teaspoons Italian
Seasoning (page xiv) or
dried oregano

¼ teaspoon crushed hot
red pepper

6 tablespoons freshly
grated Parmesan cheese
(optional)

the meatballs and sauce among six bowls, sprinkle each with 1 tablespoon of the Parmesan (if using), and serve hot.

NUTRITIONAL ANALYSIS

(1 serving: 3 meatballs with sauce) 240 calories, 22 g protein, 16 g carbohydrates, 10 g fat, 4 g fiber, 70 mg cholesterol, 513 mg sodium, 596 potassium. Food groups: ½ whole grain, 3 ounces meat, 1 vegetable, 1 fat.

Pasta and Parmesan

Everyone loves pasta…but perhaps we eat too much of it, or at least, more than we can burn off with our daily activity. The next time you're about to dig into a big bowl of spaghetti topped with a thick layer of Parmesan cheese, consider these figures:

For pasta, ¼ cup of uncooked pasta shapes (such as ziti or penne) will make ½ cup of cooked pasta. Without salt in the water, this will yield 105 calories, 4 g protein, 21 g carbohydrates, 0 g fat, 1 g fiber, 2 mg sodium, and 38 mg potassium. If you have this amount of pasta, allow 1 grain serving in your DASH calculation.

Each tablespoon of shredded natural Parmesan cheese (true Parmigiano-Reggiano or domestic Parmesan, as opposed to shelf-stable, pre-grated faux Parmesan cheese) has 21 calories, 2 g protein, 0 g carbohydrates, 2 g fat, 0 g fiber, 4 mg cholesterol, 76 mg sodium, and 5 mg potassium. But there is a lot of flavor in each tablespoon. Parmesan cheese keeps well (wrapped in foil in the refrigerator), so it is good to have on hand to use in moderation.

Cajun Turkey Burgers with Pickled Red Onions

These burgers are so juicy and flavorful that you won't need a condiment; the pickled onions are sufficient. (Refrigerate any leftover onions for up to 3 days to add to sandwiches and salads.) However, for a quick remoulade, mix ¼ cup low-fat mayonnaise, 1 teaspoon Dijon mustard, and 1 tablespoon low-sodium pickle relish. MAKES 4 SERVINGS

Pickled Red Onions

1 small red onion, cut into thin half-moons

½ cup cider vinegar, as needed

Turkey Burgers

2 teaspoons canola oil, plus more in a pump sprayer

2 celery ribs, finely chopped

½ cup finely chopped red bell pepper

2 cloves garlic, finely chopped

2 scallions, white and green parts, finely chopped

1 teaspoon Cajun Seasoning (page xiii)

1¼ pounds ground turkey

½ teaspoon kosher salt

4 whole-wheat hamburger buns, toasted

4 tomato slices

4 red lettuce leaves

To pickle the onions: Put the onions in a small bowl and add enough vinegar to cover the onions. Let stand at room temperature for at least 30 minutes and up to 6 hours.

To make the turkey burgers: Heat the 2 teaspoons oil in a large nonstick skillet over medium heat. Add the celery, bell pepper, and garlic and cook, stirring occasionally, until tender, about 5 minutes. Add the scallions and cook until wilted, about 2 minutes. Stir in the Cajun Seasoning. Transfer to a large bowl and let cool.

Add the ground turkey and salt to the vegetable mixture and combine thoroughly. Shape into four 3½-inch burgers. Place on a waxed paper–lined plate and refrigerate for 15 to 30 minutes.

Wipe out the skillet with paper towels. Spray the skillet with the oil and heat over medium heat. Add the burgers and cook until the undersides are golden brown, about 5 minutes. Flip the burgers and cook until the other sides are browned and the burgers feel resilient when pressed on top with a finger, about 5 minutes more. Remove from the skillet.

For each serving, place a burger in a bun and top with some red onions, a tomato, and a lettuce leaf. Serve hot.

NUTRITIONAL ANALYSIS

(1 serving, with a bun) 420 calories, 33 g protein, 36 g carbohydrates, 17 g fat, 6 g fiber, 105 mg cholesterol, 698 mg sodium, 698 mg potassium. Food groups: 2 whole grains, 4 ounces meat, ½ vegetable.

(1 serving, without a bun) 269 calories, 28 g protein, 7 g carbohydrates, 14 g fat, 2 g fiber, 105 mg cholesterol, 427 mg sodium, 545 mg potassium. Food groups: 4 ounces meat, ½ vegetable.

Turkey Mini Meat Loaf with Dijon Glaze

Meat loaf gets a delicious makeover with this updated version using lean ground turkey, healthful vegetables, oatmeal, and a sweet-piquant mustard glaze. This recipe is a good example of how to take a standard dish and load it with vegetables and whole grains to pump up its nutrition. Shaping the turkey mixture into individual loaves cuts down on the baking time, too.

MAKES 4 SERVINGS

2 teaspoons canola oil, plus more in a pump sprayer

1 medium yellow onion, finely chopped

1 medium carrot, cut into ¼-inch dice

1 medium celery stalk, cut into ¼-inch dice

1 tablespoon water

1¼ pounds ground turkey

¾ cup old-fashioned (rolled) oats

1 large egg, beaten

1 teaspoon dried rosemary

½ teaspoon kosher salt

¼ teaspoon freshly ground black pepper

1 tablespoon Dijon mustard

1 tablespoon honey

Preheat the oven to 350°F. Line a large baking sheet with aluminum foil and spray with oil.

Heat the 2 teaspoons oil in a medium nonstick skillet over medium heat. Add the onion, carrot, celery, and water. Cook, stirring occasionally, until the vegetables are tender, about 10 minutes. Transfer to a medium bowl and let cool slightly.

Add the ground turkey, oats, egg, rosemary, salt, and pepper and mix gently but thoroughly until combined. Divide into four equal portions and shape each on the prepared baking sheet, about 2 inches apart, into a 5 × 3-inch loaf.

Bake until lightly browned and an instant-read thermometer inserted in the center of a loaf reads about 160°F, about 35 minutes. Remove from the oven. Mix the mustard and honey in a small bowl, then spread the top of each loaf with one-quarter of the mustard mixture. Return to the oven and continue baking until the mustard mixture is glazed, about 5 minutes more. Let stand at room temperature for 5 minutes before serving.

NUTRITIONAL ANALYSIS

(1 serving) 335 calories, 32 g protein, 21 g carbohydrates, 15 g fat, 3 g fiber, 147 mg cholesterol, 484 mg sodium, 193 mg potassium. Food groups: 4½ ounces meat, 1 whole grain, 1 vegetable, 2 fats.

NOTE: If you need to restrict sodium further, eliminate the kosher salt. The fat content (and calories) of your turkey loaf will be much lower than shown in the nutritional analysis, since much of the fat will drip off the loaf.

Seafood

Busy cooks love fish and shellfish because they must be cooked quickly—if you take much more than 20 minutes to cook them, something is wrong! And there is more good news: Salmon and other fatty fish are rich in omega-3 fatty acids, whose nutritional benefits are well-known. Many people love fish, so serve this healthy protein-rich food at least three times a week. Most supermarkets now carry a large selection of fish fillets beyond the once ubiquitous flounder, so give something new a try. Most of the fish selected for each of the recipes in this section are interchangeable. Unfortunately, shellfish is on the salty side, so keep an eye on your intake, and be sure to serve a small amount with lots of vegetables to limit the sodium. That being said, it can be a lifesaver to keep a bag of individually frozen shrimp in the freezer for that occasional quick meal.

———————

Spicy Cajun Catfish Bake

The spicy flavors of Cajun dishes are perfect for low-salt cooking. Along with the traditional bell peppers, scallions, and garlic, I've added potatoes to create a one-dish meal.

MAKES 4 SERVINGS

1 tablespoon olive oil, plus more in a pump sprayer

2 medium Yukon Gold potatoes (8 ounces), scrubbed, unpeeled, and cut into ½-inch-thick slices

1 large red bell pepper, cored and cut into ½-inch dice

2 celery ribs, coarsely chopped

2 cloves garlic, coarsely chopped

2 plum (Roma) tomatoes, seeded and cut into ½-inch dice

3 scallions, white and green parts, chopped

½ teaspoon kosher salt

4 (5-ounce) catfish fillets

4 thin lemon slices, plus lemon wedges for serving

2 teaspoons Cajun Seasoning (page xiii)

Preheat the oven to 400°F. Spray a 9 × 13-inch baking dish with oil.

Heat the 1 tablespoon oil in a large nonstick skillet over medium-high heat. Add the potatoes and cook, stirring occasionally, until they begin to soften, about 5 minutes. Add the bell pepper, celery, and garlic and sauté until the pepper softens, about 5 minutes more. Stir in the tomatoes and scallions and sprinkle with the salt. Spread in the baking dish.

Bake, stirring occasionally, until the potatoes are almost tender, about 25 minutes. Remove from the oven. Arrange the catfish on the vegetable mixture and top each fillet with a lemon slice. Sprinkle the fish and vegetables with the Cajun Seasoning. Return to the oven and bake until the catfish is opaque when flaked with the tip of a knife, 8 to 10 minutes. Serve hot, with the lemon wedges.

NUTRITIONAL ANALYSIS

(1 serving) 282 calories, 24 g protein, 18 g carbohydrates, 12 g fat, 4 g fiber, 78 mg cholesterol, 412 mg sodium, 1,024 mg potassium. Food groups: 3½ ounces meat, 1 starchy vegetable, 2 vegetables, 1 fat.

Cod with Grapefruit, Avocado, and Fennel Salad

Although this dish is very simple, it has a sophisticated look that you would expect to find in a restaurant. Fennel has crunch and a mild anise flavor that can be adjusted by the amount of chopped green fronds you add to the salad. **MAKES 4 SERVINGS**

Grapefruit, Avocado, and Fennel Salad

1 small fennel bulb

2 tablespoons fresh lemon juice

1 tablespoon extra-virgin olive oil

¼ teaspoon kosher salt

¼ teaspoon freshly ground black pepper

1 ripe avocado, pitted, peeled, and cut into ½-inch dice

1 pink or red grapefruit, peel removed, cut between the membranes into segments

Cod

2 teaspoons olive oil

4 (5-ounce) cod fillets

To make the salad: Cut the fennel in half lengthwise. If the fronds are attached, cut them off and reserve. Cut out and discard the triangular core at the base of the bulb. Cut one fennel half crosswise into thin half-moons. Reserve the remaining fennel half and stalks for another use.

In a medium bowl, whisk together the lemon juice and oil, and season with salt and pepper. Add the fennel, avocado, and grapefruit and mix gently. Set aside while preparing the cod.

To prepare the cod: Heat the oil in a large nonstick skillet over medium heat. Add the cod and cover. Cook until the undersides are golden, about 3 minutes. Turn and cook, uncovered, adjusting the heat as needed, until the other side of each fillet is golden brown and the cod looks barely opaque when flaked in the center with the tip of a knife, about 3 minutes more.

Divide the fennel salad among four dinner plates. Top each with a cod fillet and serve immediately.

NUTRITIONAL ANALYSIS
(1 serving) 270 calories, 27 g protein, 14 g carbohydrates, 12 g fat, 5 g fiber, 62 mg cholesterol, 232 mg sodium, 504 mg potassium. Food groups: 4 ounces meat, 1 vegetable, ½ fruit, 1 fat.

Brown Rice Paella with Cod, Shrimp, and Asparagus

Paella can be a complicated affair, but in this streamlined version, a tight ingredient list touches all of the bases without compromising taste. If you wish, add 1 teaspoon of kosher salt to the brown rice mixture, but a squeeze of lemon may be enough to balance the flavor without salt.   MAKES 6 SERVINGS

8 ounces asparagus, woody stems discarded, cut into 1-inch lengths

1 tablespoon olive oil

1 medium yellow onion, chopped

1 medium red bell pepper, cored and cut into ½-inch dice

2 cloves garlic, minced

1 cup brown rice

2 cups Homemade Chicken Broth (page 38) or canned low-sodium chicken broth

1 (14.5-ounce) can no-salt-added diced tomatoes, drained

½ cup water

1 teaspoon dried oregano

½ teaspoon crushed hot red pepper

¼ teaspoon crushed saffron threads

12 ounces cod fillets, cut into 1-inch pieces

8 ounces large shrimp (21 to 25), peeled and deveined

Lemon wedges, for serving

Bring a small saucepan of water to a boil over high heat. Add the asparagus and cook until crisp and bright green, about 2 minutes. (It will finish cooking later.) Drain, rinse under cold running water, and drain again. Set aside.

Heat the oil in a medium Dutch oven or flameproof casserole over medium heat. Add the onion, bell pepper, and garlic and cook, stirring occasionally, until softened, about 3 minutes. Stir in the brown rice. Add the broth, tomatoes, water, oregano, hot pepper, and saffron and bring to a boil. Reduce the heat to medium-low and simmer, covered, until the rice has almost completely absorbed the liquid, about 40 minutes.

Add the cod, shrimp, and asparagus to the Dutch oven. Cover and cook until the cod is opaque throughout, about 5 minutes. Remove from the heat and uncover. Let stand for 3 minutes. Serve hot, with the lemon wedges.

NUTRITIONAL ANALYSIS
(1 serving) 266 calories, 21 g protein, 35 g carbohydrates, 5 g fat, 4 g fiber, 73 mg cholesterol, 302 mg sodium, 365 mg potassium. Food groups: 3 ounces meat, 2 whole grains, 1 vegetable.

Fish Tacos with Lime-Cilantro Slaw

Fish tacos make a family-friendly meal that can be cooked in minutes. This version has a slaw that is made even easier with coleslaw mix—no shredding necessary. Remember that if you want to save some calories, serve the fish mixture in Bibb or romaine lettuce leaves instead of tortillas. **MAKES 6 SERVINGS**

Fish

2 tablespoons fresh lime juice

2 teaspoons chili powder

1½ pounds cod fillets

Slaw

Freshly grated zest of 1 lime

2 tablespoons fresh lime juice

2 tablespoons light mayonnaise

1 (12-ounce) bag coleslaw mix

2 plum (Roma) tomatoes, seeded and cut into ½-inch dice

2 scallions, white and green parts, finely chopped

2 tablespoons finely chopped fresh cilantro

½ teaspoon kosher salt

Olive oil in a pump sprayer

12 (6-inch) corn tortillas, warmed

Lime wedges, for serving

To prepare the fish: Whisk together the lime juice and chili powder in a shallow glass or ceramic baking dish. Add the cod and turn to coat. Cover and refrigerate while making the slaw.

To make the slaw: In a large bowl, whisk together the lime zest and juice and mayonnaise. Add the coleslaw mix, tomatoes, scallions, cilantro, and salt and mix well. Set aside.

Spray a large nonstick skillet with oil and heat over medium-high heat. Remove the fish from the baking dish, letting the excess juice drip back into the dish. Place in the skillet and cook, turning occasionally, until opaque when flaked in the thickest part with the tip of a knife, about 8 minutes. Transfer to a serving bowl and flake into large chunks with a fork.

For each serving, spoon some fish and slaw on a tortilla, then fold and eat, with a squeeze of lime juice, if you wish.

NUTRITIONAL ANALYSIS

(1 serving) 247 calories, 24 g protein, 29 g carbohydrates, 4 g fat, 6 g fiber, 51 mg cholesterol, 308 mg sodium, 236 mg potassium. Food groups: 3 ounces meat, 2 whole grains, 1 vegetable.

Halibut with Spring Vegetables

This elegant dish of poached halibut and vegetables is reminiscent of something you might order at an upscale restaurant. Feel free to add your favorite vegetables to the skillet with the halibut. Asparagus spears, sugar snap peas, or peas would all be welcome.

MAKES 4 SERVINGS

8 baby red-skinned potatoes (about 1 ounce each), scrubbed but unpeeled, cut in halves

32 baby carrots, preferably not baby-cut carrots, trimmed

1 tablespoon unsalted butter

1 cup chopped leeks, white and pale green parts only

1 cup Homemade Chicken Broth (page 38) or canned low-sodium chicken broth

½ cup water

¼ cup dry vermouth or white wine

4 (5-ounce) skinless halibut fillets

¼ teaspoon kosher salt

¼ teaspoon freshly ground black pepper

Finely chopped fresh chives, parsley, or a combination, for serving

Lemon wedges, for serving

Bring a medium saucepan of water to a boil over high heat. Add the potatoes, reduce heat to medium, and cook at a steady simmer for 5 minutes. Add the carrots and cook until the vegetables are almost, but not quite, tender when pierced with the tip of a small, sharp knife, about 3 minutes more. Drain and rinse under cold running water.

Melt the butter in a large skillet over medium heat. Add the leeks and cover. Cook, stirring occasionally, until tender, about 5 minutes. Add the broth, water, and vermouth and bring to a simmer. Reduce the heat to medium-low, cover partially with the lid, and simmer for 5 minutes to blend the flavors.

Spread the potatoes and carrots in the skillet in a single layer. Arrange the halibut fillets on the vegetables and season with the salt and pepper. Cover tightly and simmer until the vegetables are tender and the halibut is opaque in the center when pierced with the tip of a small, sharp knife, 10 to 12 minutes.

Divide the vegetables and broth evenly among four deep soup bowls. Top each with a halibut fillet and sprinkle with the herbs. Add the lemon wedges and serve hot.

NUTRITIONAL ANALYSIS
(1 serving) 256 calories, 29 g protein, 19 g carbohydrates, 5 g fat, 4 g fiber, 77 mg cholesterol, 270 mg sodium, 1,170 mg potassium. Food groups: 4 ounces meat, 1 starchy vegetable, 1 vegetable.

Roasted Salmon Fillets with Basil Drizzle

This is a basic recipe for quickly roasting salmon fillets, which are drizzled with a basil puree just before serving. You could consider roasting extra fillets to press into service for the Salmon *Salade Niçoise* and the Salmon and Edamame Cakes on pages 52 and 135. I like to serve these with the Broccoli Rabe with Pine Nuts (page 164).   MAKES 4 SERVINGS

Salmon

Olive oil in a pump sprayer

4 (6-ounce) skinless salmon fillets

¼ teaspoon kosher salt

¼ teaspoon freshly ground black pepper

Basil Drizzle

1 clove garlic, peeled

½ cup packed fresh basil leaves

3 tablespoons coarsely chopped fresh parsley leaves

2 tablespoons water

1 tablespoon balsamic vinegar

Pinch of kosher salt

Pinch of freshly ground black pepper

¼ cup extra-virgin olive oil

To prepare the salmon: Preheat the oven to 400°F. Spray a 9 × 13-inch baking dish with oil.

Place the salmon fillets in the baking dish, spray with oil, and season with the salt and pepper. Roast until the salmon looks barely opaque when prodded in the thickest part with the tip of a knife, about 10 minutes.

Meanwhile, make the basil drizzle: With a food processor running, drop the garlic clove through the feed tube to mince the garlic. (Or drop the garlic through the hole in the lid of a blender.) Stop the food processor or blender, add the basil, parsley, water, vinegar, salt, and pepper, and pulse a few times to chop the herbs. With the motor running, gradually add the oil. Pour the drizzle mixture into a small bowl.

Using a metal spatula, transfer the fillets to dinner plates and drizzle with equal amounts of the basil mixture. Serve hot.

NUTRITIONAL ANALYSIS
(1 serving: 1 [6-ounce] fillet) 370 calories, 34 g protein, 1 g carbohydrates, 24 g fat, 0 g fiber, 94 mg cholesterol, 250 mg sodium, 895 mg potassium. Food groups: 5 ounces meat.

(For a smaller appetite: 1 [3-ounce] serving) 247 calories, 23 g protein, 1 g carbohydrates, 16 g fat, 0 g fiber, 62 mg cholesterol, 167 mg sodium, 583 mg potassium. Food groups: 3 ounces meat.

Salmon and Edamame Cakes

When you have lemons, make lemonade. And when you have cooked salmon, make salmon cakes. These are seasoned Asian-style with ginger, scallion, and cilantro and need no more than a squirt of lime juice to finish them off. They are especially tasty served with the Asian Slaw with Ginger Dressing on page 63.   MAKES 4 SERVINGS

2 cups flaked cooked salmon (about 13 ounces), such as Roasted Salmon Fillets with Basil Drizzle (page 134)

¼ cup panko (Japanese-style bread crumbs), preferably whole-wheat panko (see page 140)

2 large egg whites

1 tablespoon peeled and minced fresh ginger

1 scallion, white and green parts, finely chopped

1 tablespoon finely chopped fresh cilantro

1 clove garlic, crushed through a press

½ cup thawed frozen edamame

Canola oil in a pump sprayer

Lime wedges, for serving

In a medium bowl, mix the salmon, panko, egg whites, ginger, scallion, cilantro, and garlic. Stir in the edamame. Shape the mixture into four 3½-inch-wide cakes. Transfer to a waxed paper–lined plate and refrigerate for 15 to 30 minutes.

Spray a large nonstick skillet with oil and heat over medium heat. Add the salmon cakes and cook until the undersides are browned, 3 to 4 minutes. Flip the cakes over and cook until the other sides are browned, 3 to 4 minutes more. Serve hot, with the lime wedges.

NUTRITIONAL ANALYSIS

(1 serving) 267 calories, 21 g protein, 5 g carbohydrates, 13 g fat, 1 g fiber, 47 mg cholesterol, 166 mg sodium, 556 mg potassium. Food groups: 3 ounces meat, ¼ grain, 1 fat.

Sea Scallops and Vegetables with Ginger Sauce

Chinese cooks have a culinary trick called velveting. The meat (or in this case, seafood) is par-cooked before it is stir-fried to give it a smooth, velvety texture. It takes only a minute, so give it a try. Here I use the technique with tender scallops before they are stir-fried with brightly colored vegetables. Serve this with ½ cup cooked Basic Brown Rice (page 174) if you wish.   MAKES 4 SERVINGS

1 pound sea scallops, each cut in half horizontally

¾ cup low-sodium chicken broth

1 tablespoon reduced-sodium soy sauce

1 tablespoon rice vinegar

¼ teaspoon crushed hot red pepper

2 teaspoons cornstarch

1 tablespoon canola or vegetable oil

8 ounces sugar snap peas, trimmed

1 large red bell pepper, cored and cut into 2 × ¼-inch strips

2 scallions, white and green parts, 1 minced and 1 finely chopped

1½ tablespoons peeled and minced fresh ginger

2 cloves garlic, minced

Bring a medium saucepan of water to a boil over high heat. Add the scallops and cook just until they turn opaque around the edges, about 30 seconds. Drain.

In a glass measuring cup, combine the broth, soy sauce, vinegar, and hot pepper. Sprinkle in the cornstarch and stir with a fork until dissolved. Set aside.

Heat a large wok or skillet over high heat. Drizzle in the oil, tilting the wok to coat the entire surface. Add the sugar snap peas and bell pepper and stir-fry until beginning to soften, about 1 minute. Stir in the minced scallion, ginger, and garlic and stir-fry until fragrant, about 30 seconds. Add the scallops and broth mixture and bring to a boil, stirring often. Cook until the scallops are opaque throughout and the sauce is thickened, about 1 minute.

Divide the scallop mixture evenly among four bowls, sprinkle with the chopped scallion, and serve hot.

NUTRITIONAL ANALYSIS

(1 serving) 169 calories, 17 g protein, 14 g carbohydrates, 4 g fat, 3 g fiber, 27 mg cholesterol, 763 mg sodium, 516 mg potassium. Food groups: 3 ounces meat, 1 vegetable.

Shrimp with Corn Hash

A trip to the farmer's market in summer inspired this dish, which is ready in minutes. Feel free to use thawed frozen corn kernels instead of fresh. The lemon and basil will season this nicely, so hold off on the salt, as shrimp is naturally high in sodium.

MAKES 4 SERVINGS

4 teaspoons olive oil

1 pound large shrimp (21 to 25), peeled and deveined

½ cup chopped red onion

½ medium red bell pepper, seeded and cut into ½-inch dice

1½ cups fresh corn kernels, cut from 2 large ears of corn

1 cup halved cherry or grape tomatoes

¼ teaspoon crushed hot red pepper

¼ cup water

1 tablespoon fresh lemon juice

2 tablespoons coarsely chopped fresh basil

Heat 2 teaspoons of the oil in a large nonstick skillet over medium-high heat. Add the shrimp and cook, stirring occasionally, until it is opaque throughout, 3 to 5 minutes. Transfer to a plate.

Heat the remaining 2 teaspoons oil in the skillet over medium-high heat. Add the onion and bell pepper and cook, stirring often, until softened, about 1 minute. Add the corn, tomatoes, and hot pepper and cover. Cook, stirring occasionally, until these vegetables are heated through, about 3 minutes.

Add the shrimp and reheat, stirring often, about 1 minute. Stir in the water and lemon juice and cook, scraping up any browned bits in the pan with a wooden spoon. Transfer to a serving bowl and sprinkle with the basil. Serve hot.

NUTRITIONAL ANALYSIS
(1 serving) 195 calories, 18 g protein, 18 g carbohydrates, 6 g fat, 3 g fiber, 142 mg cholesterol, 647 mg sodium, 420 mg potassium. Food groups: 3 ounces meat, 1 whole grain, 1 vegetable.

Greek Shrimp with Zucchini and Grape Tomatoes

Greek cooks often combine shrimp, tomatoes, and oregano, and I've added zucchini to increase the vegetable content. Most of the sodium in this recipe comes from the shrimp, so keep an eye on your sodium intake for the day if you have this for dinner. I've omitted added-salt entirely to let the goat cheese provide the seasoning.　　MAKES 4 SERVINGS

3 teaspoons olive oil

1 pound large shrimp (21 to 25), peeled and deveined

1 large zucchini, halved lengthwise and cut into ¼-inch-thick half-moons

2 tablespoons minced shallot

1 clove garlic, minced

1 pint grape or cherry tomatoes, halved lengthwise

¼ teaspoon freshly ground black pepper

2 tablespoons dry vermouth

Grated zest of 1 lemon

2 tablespoons fresh lemon juice

1 tablespoon finely chopped fresh oregano, or 1 teaspoon dried oregano

¼ cup (1 ounce) crumbled goat cheese, for serving

Heat 1 teaspoon of the oil in a large nonstick skillet over medium-high heat. Add the shrimp and cook, stirring occasionally, until it turns opaque, about 3 minutes. The shrimp will be slightly undercooked at this point. Transfer to a plate.

Heat the remaining 2 teaspoons oil in the skillet. Add the zucchini and sauté, stirring occasionally, until crisp-tender and lightly browned, about 5 minutes. Stir in the shallot and garlic and cook until they are fragrant, about 30 seconds. Add the tomatoes and pepper and cook, stirring often, until heated through, about 3 minutes.

Return the shrimp to the skillet and add the vermouth, lemon zest and juice, and oregano. Cook, stirring often, to reheat the shrimp, about 1 minute.

Transfer to a serving bowl and top with the goat cheese. Serve hot.

NUTRITIONAL ANALYSIS
(1 serving) 184 calories, 22 g protein, 10 g carbohydrates, 6 g fat, 3 g fiber, 180 mg cholesterol, 823 mg sodium, 625 mg potassium. Food groups: 3 ounces meat, ½ vegetable.

Crispy Tilapia with Mediterranean Vegetables

Let the oven do most of the work for this healthful entrée of fresh seafood on a bed of vegetables. Use an ovenproof skillet to par-cook the vegetables, and this becomes a one-dish meal. MAKES 4 SERVINGS

1 tablespoon olive oil, plus more in a pump sprayer

1 medium yellow onion, chopped

2 cloves garlic, minced

1 medium zucchini, cut in half lengthwise and then into ½-inch-thick slices

1 medium yellow squash, cut in half lengthwise and then into ½-inch-thick slices

4 plum (Roma) tomatoes, seeded and cut into ½-inch dice

Freshly grated zest of 1 lemon

2 tablespoons fresh lemon juice

1 tablespoon chopped fresh oregano, or 1 teaspoon dried oregano

¼ teaspoon crushed hot red pepper

4 (5-ounce) tilapia fillets

3 tablespoons panko (Japanese-style bread crumbs), preferably whole-wheat panko (see page 140)

Preheat the oven to 350°F.

Heat the 1 tablespoon oil in a large ovenproof nonstick skillet over medium heat. Add the onion and garlic and cook, stirring occasionally, until softened, about 3 minutes. Add the zucchini and yellow squash and cook until softened, about 3 minutes. Stir in the tomatoes, lemon zest and juice, oregano, and hot pepper. Remove from the heat. Arrange the tilapia fillets on the vegetables. Sprinkle with the panko and spray with oil.

Bake until the tilapia is opaque when flaked in the thickest part with the tip of a knife, about 12 minutes. Serve hot.

NUTRITIONAL ANALYSIS

(1 serving) 240 calories, 32 g protein, 16 g carbohydrates, 6 g fat, 4 g fiber, 71 mg cholesterol, 96 mg sodium, 1,018 mg potassium. Food groups: 4½ ounces meat, ½ grain, 2 vegetables.

Panko

Panko, extra-crisp Japanese bread crumbs, used to be an exotic Japanese ingredient, but now it has gone mainstream and you can even buy it in various flavors. It adds crunchy texture to many dishes and is a nice topping for fish fillets. Use whole-wheat panko if you can find it, because it has a slightly better nutritional profile and less sodium than plain panko. Ian's Panko is a good brand that is sold at many natural food markets.

You can make your own coarse bread crumbs as a substitute. Lightly toast a slice of whole-wheat bread and let it cool. Tear the bread into a few pieces and process in a blender or food processor until you have coarse crumbs. When the bread crumbs are spread on food as a topping, spray the crumbs lightly with olive or canola oil from a pump-style sprayer.

Tuna with Fennel and Potatoes

Fennel (sometimes called anise) should be as popular with cooks in America as it is in Italy. Admittedly, it has a licorice flavor when raw, but the taste is milder when it is cooked. If the fronds (or leaves) have already been removed from the fennel when you buy it, you can substitute chopped fresh oregano, basil or tarragon, or parsley. A touch of Parmesan cheese brings out the flavors of the vegetables in this recipe.   MAKES 4 SERVINGS

Vegetables

1 tablespoon olive oil, plus more in a pump sprayer

1 head fennel (about 1 pound)

3 medium potatoes, scrubbed but unpeeled, cut in halves and then crosswise into ¼-inch-thick slices

1 large red bell pepper, cored and cut into ¼-inch-wide strips

4 cloves garlic, chopped

Freshly grated zest of 1 lemon

1 teaspoon kosher salt

½ teaspoon crushed hot red pepper

2 tablespoons freshly grated Parmesan cheese

Tuna

Olive oil in a pump sprayer

4 (6-ounce) tuna steaks, about 1 inch thick

½ teaspoon freshly ground black pepper

Lemon wedges, for serving

Preheat the oven to 400°F.

To prepare the vegetables: Spray a 9 × 13-inch baking dish with oil. Cut the fronds (leaves) off the fennel. Chop 2 tablespoons of fennel fronds and reserve. Cut the fennel head in half lengthwise, and cut out the thick triangular core at the bottom of the head. Cut the head and stalks crosswise into ¼- to ½-inch-wide strips.

Heat the 1 tablespoon oil in a large nonstick skillet over medium-high heat. Add the potatoes and cook, stirring occasionally, until they begin to soften around the edges, about 5 minutes. Stir in the fennel, bell pepper, garlic, lemon zest, salt, and hot pepper. Spread in the baking dish. Bake, stirring occasionally, until the potatoes are tender, about 30 minutes. During the last 5 minutes, sprinkle with the Parmesan. Remove from the oven and let stand while preparing the tuna.

To prepare the tuna: Wipe the skillet clean with paper towels. Spray the skillet with oil and heat over medium-high heat. Season the tuna with the pepper. Place the tuna steaks in the skillet and cook until the undersides are seared, about 2 minutes. Flip the tuna and cook until the other sides are seared, about 2 minutes more for rare tuna.

Divide the vegetables equally among four dinner plates, and top each with a tuna steak. Sprinkle with the reserved chopped fronds. Serve hot, with the lemon wedges.

NUTRITIONAL ANALYSIS
(1 serving) 335 calories, 40 g protein, 29 g carbohydrates, 5 g fat, 7 g fiber, 75 mg cholesterol, 372 mg sodium, 960 mg potassium. Food groups: 5 ounces meat, 1 starchy vegetable, 1 vegetable.

(1 serving [4 ounces tuna], for a smaller appetite): 223 calories, 27 g protein, 19 g carbohydrates, 4 g fat, 5 g fiber, 50 mg cholesterol, 248 mg sodium, 640 mg potassium. Food groups: 3½ ounces meat, ½ starchy vegetable, 1 vegetable.

——Vegetarian Main—— Courses

———

I've had many vegetarian students and a good number of clients who don't eat meat. Although I am a card-carrying omnivore, I often cook meatless meals that were developed with my students, to add variety to my own menus. If you cook for vegetable haters, one way to get them to eat their veggies is to add them to popular dishes like chili and macaroni and cheese. Try my recipes for these two comfort food stalwarts, and I will be very surprised if you hear complaints from the meat lovers—and the same goes for the other dishes in this chapter.

———

Cauliflower Macaroni and Cheese

This is the quintessential family-friendly DASH meal. Instead of macaroni alone, add lots of cauliflower, a "supervegetable" of the Brassicaceae family that is loaded with phytochemicals, vitamins, and minerals. Another trick here is to combine Cheddar cheese with naturally low-sodium Swiss cheese, which pumps up the flavor and reduces the sodium. Want to further boost the DASH factor with extra veggies? Layer sliced tomatoes on the cauliflower mixture, then sprinkle the panko on top.   MAKES 8 SERVINGS

1 head cauliflower, trimmed and broken into bite-sized florets

1¼ cups elbow macaroni

Canola oil in a pump sprayer

2 cups low-fat (1%) milk

1 tablespoon cornstarch

1 teaspoon dry mustard powder

4 ounces (1 cup) shredded reduced-sodium mild Cheddar cheese

4 ounces (1 cup) shredded Swiss cheese

¼ teaspoon freshly ground black pepper

¼ cup panko (Japanese-style bread crumbs), preferably whole-wheat panko (see page 140)

Bring a large pot of water to a boil over high heat. Add the cauliflower and cook just until crisp-tender, about 5 minutes. Using a wire sieve or a skimmer, transfer the cauliflower to a colander; leave the water boiling. Drain well. Pat the cauliflower dry with paper towels.

Add the macaroni to the boiling water and cook according to the package directions until it is almost tender, about 7 minutes. Drain well.

Preheat the oven to 350°F. Spray a 9 × 13-inch baking dish with oil.

Pour the milk into a medium saucepan. Sprinkle in the cornstarch and mustard and whisk to dissolve the cornstarch. Bring to a boil over medium heat, whisking often to avoid scorching; the sauce will thicken when it comes to a boil. Remove from the heat, add the cheeses and pepper, and whisk until smooth. Add the cauliflower and macaroni and mix well. Spread in the baking dish and sprinkle with the panko.

Bake until the sauce is bubbling, about 20 minutes. Let stand at room temperature for 5 minutes, then serve hot.

NUTRITIONAL ANALYSIS
(1 serving) 234 calories, 13 g protein, 23 g carbohydrates, 10 g fat, 2 g fiber, 30 mg cholesterol, 88 mg sodium, 405 mg potassium. Food groups: 1 grain, 1 dairy, 1 vegetable.

Roasted Eggplant Parmesan

Traditional eggplant Parmesan is made with fried eggplant and loads of cheese, both of which can pile up the calories. Some cooks salt eggplant to draw out bitter juices, but this is unnecessary with modern varieties. This lightened-up recipe—high in fiber, rich in potassium—roasts the eggplant, uses just enough reduced-sodium mozzarella, and gets a blast of flavor from fresh basil. You can use store-bought low-sodium marinara sauce instead of the homemade, but the sodium numbers will go up.   MAKES 6 SERVINGS

Olive oil in a pump sprayer

2 (1¾-pound) eggplants, trimmed and cut crosswise into 24 (½-inch-thick) rounds

3 cups Marinara Sauce (see page 147)

1 cup (4 ounces) shredded low-sodium mozzarella

¼ cup (1 ounce) freshly grated Parmesan cheese

½ cup packed chopped fresh basil, for serving

Position racks in the top third and center of the oven and preheat the oven to 400°F. Line two large baking sheets with parchment paper. Spray the paper with oil.

Arrange the eggplant slices on the baking sheets (they can be crowded). Spray the tops of the slices with the oil. Roast until the eggplant is lightly browned, 10 to 15 minutes. Flip the slices over and cook until the eggplant is tender, about 15 minutes more. Let cool until easy to handle.

Reduce the oven temperature to 350°F. Lightly spray a 9 × 13-inch baking dish with oil. Spread about ½ cup of the sauce in the bottom of the pan. Top with half of the eggplant slices (they can be crowded) and sprinkle with the mozzarella. Top with the remaining eggplant. Spread the remaining sauce over the eggplant and sprinkle with the Parmesan.

Bake until the sauce is bubbling and the Parmesan is lightly browned, about 20 minutes. Let cool for 5 minutes. Serve the eggplant, topping each serving with a generous sprinkle of basil.

NUTRITIONAL ANALYSIS
(1 serving) 144 calories, 9 g protein, 20 g carbohydrates, 5 g fat, 10 g fiber, 10 mg cholesterol, 165 mg sodium, 637 mg potassium. Food groups: 2 vegetables, 1 dairy.

Marinara Sauce

Pasta sauce is another item you can get in a low-sodium form, but homemade is so much tastier and is made without added chemicals. Although you won't find carrots and celery in every marinara sauce recipe, I add them to mine to increase the vegetables and sweeten the sauce naturally. This is a great recipe to freeze in 2-cup containers and use as needed. If you wish, substitute dry vermouth for the balsamic vinegar.

MAKES 1 QUART

---

1 tablespoon olive oil

1 medium onion, finely chopped

2 medium carrots, finely chopped

2 medium celery ribs, finely chopped

1 clove garlic, minced

1 (28-ounce) can no-salt-added crushed tomatoes

¾ cup water

2 tablespoons balsamic vinegar

2 teaspoons Italian Seasoning (page xiv)

1 bay leaf

Heat the oil in a medium saucepan over medium heat. Add the onion, carrots, celery, and garlic and cover. Cook, stirring occasionally, until tender, about 6 minutes. Stir in the tomatoes, water, vinegar, Italian Seasoning, and bay leaf and bring to a simmer. Reduce the heat to medium-low, uncover, and simmer, stirring occasionally, until lightly thickened, about 1 hour. Remove the bay leaf. (The sauce can be cooled, covered, and refrigerated for up to 5 days or frozen for up to 2 months.)

NUTRITIONAL ANALYSIS
(1 serving: ½ cup) 59 calories, 1 g protein, 10 g carbohydrates, 2 g fat, 3 g fiber, 0 mg cholesterol, 61 mg sodium, 125 mg potassium. Food groups: 2 vegetables.

Bell Peppers with Rice and Vegetable Stuffing

Here is a wonderful vegetarian version of one of the all-time great comfort foods, stuffed peppers. Be sure to allow a head start to simmer the brown rice. This is the vegetarian version, and I also provide a beef variation. MAKES 4 SERVINGS

⅓ cup brown rice

1 tablespoon olive oil, plus more in a pump sprayer

4 red bell peppers

¼ cup pine nuts

1 medium yellow onion, finely chopped

2 cloves garlic, minced

1 (10-ounce) package thawed and chopped frozen spinach, squeezed to remove excess moisture

1 teaspoon Italian Seasoning (page xiv)

½ cup (2 ounces) chopped reduced-fat Swiss cheese

2 tablespoons panko (Japanese-style bread crumbs), preferably whole-wheat panko (see page 140)

1 large egg white

¼ teaspoon kosher salt

¼ teaspoon freshly ground black pepper

1 (14.5-ounce) can no-salt-added petite diced tomatoes with juice, undrained

Bring a medium saucepan of water to a boil over high heat. Add the rice and reduce the heat to medium-low. Simmer until the rice is just tender, about 40 minutes. Drain and rinse under cold running water.

Meanwhile, preheat the oven to 350°F. Spray a 9 × 13-inch baking dish with oil to lightly coat.

Cut the tops from the bell peppers to make "lids." Discard the stems and dice the pepper tops. Using a spoon, scoop out and discard the ribs and seeds from the peppers. If needed, trim the bottoms of the peppers so they can stand without tilting. Set aside.

Heat a medium skillet over medium heat. Spread the pine nuts evenly in the skillet and cook, stirring occasionally, until toasted, about 3 minutes. Transfer to a bowl.

Heat the 1 tablespoon oil in the skillet. Add the onion, diced pepper tops, and garlic and cook, stirring occasionally, until the onion is tender, about 4 minutes. Add the spinach and Italian Seasoning and stir to evaporate excess moisture, about 1 minute. Transfer to the bowl with the pine nuts and let cool slightly. Stir in the rice, cheese, panko, egg white, salt, and pepper and mix well.

Divide the spinach mixture evenly among the peppers, pressing it firmly into each to make a high mound, and then place the peppers in the baking dish. Pour the tomatoes and their juice around the peppers. Cover tightly with aluminum foil and bake for 45 minutes. Uncover and bake until the peppers are tender when pierced with the tip of a small, sharp knife, about 30 minutes more. Divide the peppers and tomatoes among four shallow bowls and serve.

NUTRITIONAL ANALYSIS
(1 serving) 276 calories, 12 g protein, 34 g carbohydrates, 11 g fat, 8 g fiber, 5 mg cholesterol, 156 mg sodium, 677 mg potassium. Food groups: 2 starches, 2 vegetables, 1 dairy, ¼ nuts.

Variation

Bell Peppers with Beef and Vegetable Stuffing: Reduce the brown rice to ¼ cup. Add 4 ounces ground sirloin to the cooked onion mixture and cook, breaking up the meat with the side of a spoon, until it loses its pink color, about 5 minutes.

NUTRITIONAL ANALYSIS
(1 serving) 297 calories, 18 g protein, 31 g carbohydrates, 12 g fat, 8 g fiber, 21 mg cholesterol, 170 mg sodium, 748 mg potassium. Food groups: 1½ starches, 1 ounce meat, 2 vegetables, 1 dairy, ¼ nuts.

Freezing Brown Rice

With white rice, the nutritious bran has been removed. Brown rice has the bran intact, to provide vitamins, fiber, and texture. The only problem with brown rice is that it takes a long time to cook, especially for a weeknight meal. This is easy to fix by cooking the brown rice ahead of time.

Simply simmer the brown rice in water until it is tender, about 45 minutes. The rice will expand during cooking to about three times its original size: 1 cup uncooked brown rice will yield about 3 cups cooked rice. Drain and rinse the rice under cold running water and let it cool completely. Store the rice in zippered plastic freezer bags and freeze for up to 3 months. When you want to serve it, just microwave in the bag until it is heated through, about 3 minutes on high for 2 cups of cooked rice.

Vegetable and Bulgur Chili

This vegetarian dish is packed with vegetables and is very filling, even though it is low in calories. Adding bulgur to vegetable chili thickens the juices to provide a meaty texture. There are many add-ins that you can stir into the pot—corn kernels, canned beans, and cubes of butternut squash are just a few. You could serve it with a half sandwich, fruit, and some yogurt for a great weekday lunch. If you are watching sodium, you can reduce the salt or eliminate it.   MAKES 8 SERVINGS

1 tablespoon olive oil

1 large yellow onion, chopped

2 medium carrots, cut into ½-inch rounds

2 medium celery ribs, cut into ½-inch slices

1 large red bell pepper, cored and cut into ½-inch pieces

1 large zucchini, cut into ½-inch-thick half-moons

3 cloves garlic, minced

1 tablespoon chili powder, or 1 canned chipotle in adobo, minced

2 cups water

1 (14.5-ounce) can no-salt-added diced tomatoes with juice, undrained

1 teaspoon kosher salt

½ cup bulgur

8 tablespoons nonfat sour cream, for serving

Chopped fresh cilantro, for serving

Lime wedges, for serving

Heat the oil in a medium Dutch oven or flameproof casserole over medium heat. Add the onion, carrots, celery, bell pepper, zucchini, and garlic. Cover and cook, stirring occasionally, until the vegetables soften, about 5 minutes. Stir in the chili powder and cook for 30 seconds.

Stir in the water, tomatoes with their juice, and salt. Bring to a simmer. Reduce the heat to low and partially cover the Dutch oven. Simmer, stirring occasionally, until the vegetables are tender, about 30 minutes.

Stir in the bulgur. Simmer until the bulgur is tender, adding more hot water as needed if the chili gets too thick, about 20 minutes more. Divide among eight soup bowls, and top each with a tablespoon of sour cream and a sprinkle of cilantro. Serve hot, with the lime wedges.

NUTRITIONAL ANALYSIS
(1 serving) 109 calories, 3 g protein, 21 g carbohydrates, 2 g fat, 5 g fiber, 1 mg cholesterol, 337 mg sodium, 342 mg potassium. Food groups: 1 whole grain, 2 vegetables.

Moroccan Vegetables on Garbanzo Couscous

With the bold flavors in this vegetable stew, the need for salt is highly reduced. I do put a little in the couscous, however. Although it's not traditional, you might like to top each serving with a dollop of yogurt to increase the protein. MAKES 6 SERVINGS

Vegetables

1 teaspoon sweet paprika, preferably Hungarian or Spanish

1 teaspoon ground coriander

1 teaspoon ground ginger

¾ teaspoon kosher salt

½ teaspoon freshly ground black pepper

¼ teaspoon cayenne

1 (1¾-pound) butternut squash, peeled, seeded, and cut into 1-inch pieces

4 large carrots, cut into ½-inch-thick rounds

2 large zucchini, cut into ½-inch-thick rounds

1 large red bell pepper, cored and cut into 1-inch squares

1 large yellow onion, unpeeled, cut into sixths

2 tablespoons olive oil

2 garlic cloves, coarsely chopped

Couscous

1 cup water

½ cup whole-wheat couscous

Continued

Preheat the oven to 400°F.

To prepare the vegetables: Mix the paprika, coriander, ginger, salt, pepper, and cayenne in a small bowl and set aside. In a large roasting pan, combine the squash, carrots, zucchini, bell pepper, and onion. Add the oil and mix gently to coat. Roast, stirring occasionally, until the vegetables are lightly browned and tender, about 1 hour. During the last 5 minutes, stir in the spice mixture and garlic.

Meanwhile, prepare the couscous: In a medium saucepan, bring the water to a boil. Remove from the heat and stir in the couscous. Immediately add the garbanzo beans and cover tightly. Let stand until the liquid is absorbed, about 5 minutes.

When the vegetables are done, transfer them to a deep serving platter. Place the roasting pan over medium heat on the stove. Add the tomato sauce and water and bring to a boil, scraping up the browned juices in the pan with a wooden spoon. Pour over the vegetables and mix gently.

Fluff the couscous mixture with a fork. Spoon the couscous into six soup bowls, top with equal amounts of the vegetable mixture, and sprinkle with cilantro. Serve hot, with the lemon wedges.

1 (15-ounce) can reduced-sodium garbanzo beans (chickpeas), drained and rinsed

1 cup no-salt-added tomato sauce

½ cup water

Chopped fresh cilantro or mint, for garnish

Lemon wedges, for serving

NUTRITIONAL ANALYSIS

(1 serving) 295 calories, 10 g protein, 56 g carbohydrates, 6 g fat, 12 g fiber, 0 mg cholesterol, 431 mg sodium, 1,213 mg potassium. Food groups: 1 beans, 2 whole grains, 3 vegetables.

Curried Vegetables and Garbanzo Beans

The intriguing flavors of Indian cuisine are in full sail in this vegetarian entrée. You could serve it on brown rice, but potatoes provide enough starch to make this filling.

MAKES 4 SERVINGS

1 tablespoon canola oil

4 medium red-skinned potatoes (about 1 pound), scrubbed but unpeeled, cut into ½-inch-thick slices

4 medium carrots, cut into ¼-inch-thick rounds

4 medium celery ribs, cut into ¼-inch-thick slices

2 medium yellow onions, cut into ¼-inch-thick half-moons

1 tablespoon curry powder

¼ teaspoon cayenne pepper

1 cup light coconut milk

½ cup water

½ cup canned reduced-sodium garbanzo beans (chickpeas), drained and rinsed

½ cup plain low-fat yogurt

Chopped fresh cilantro, for serving

Lime wedges, for serving

Heat the oil in a large nonstick skillet over medium-high heat. Add the potatoes and cook, stirring occasionally, until they begin to soften around the edges, about 5 minutes. Add the carrots, celery, and onions and cook, stirring often, until the onions soften, about 5 minutes more. Stir in the curry powder and cayenne pepper.

Stir in the coconut milk and water and bring to a simmer. Reduce the heat to medium-low and cover. Cook, stirring occasionally, until the potatoes are tender when pierced with the tip of a small, sharp knife, about 25 minutes. During the last 5 minutes, add the garbanzo beans.

To serve, divide among four soup bowls and top each with 2 tablespoons yogurt and a sprinkle of cilantro. Serve hot, with the lime wedges.

NUTRITIONAL ANALYSIS

(1 serving) 271 calories, 7 g protein, 39 g carbohydrates, 11 g fat, 8 g fiber, 2 mg cholesterol, 207 mg sodium, 1,106 mg potassium. Food groups: 1 beans, 1 starchy vegetable, 1 vegetable.

Summer Vegetable Risotto

Like pasta, risotto is a beloved Italian dish that can be enjoyed on the DASH plan when it is combined with lots of vegetables. The rice needs near constant attention, but it is fun to stand in front of the stove and stir while chatting with friends or family. Don't heap Parmesan onto the risotto; use just enough to season each serving.   MAKES 4 SERVINGS

4 teaspoons olive oil

2 medium zucchini, cut into ½-inch dice

1 medium yellow onion, chopped

1 clove garlic, minced

1 cup halved cherry or grape tomatoes

½ teaspoon kosher salt

¼ teaspoon freshly ground black pepper

2½ cups Homemade Chicken Broth (page 38) or canned low-sodium chicken broth

2½ cups water

1 cup Italian rice for risotto, such as arborio

2 tablespoons finely chopped fresh oregano

Freshly grated zest of 1 lemon

4 tablespoons freshly grated Parmesan cheese, for serving

Heat 2 teaspoons of the oil in a medium Dutch oven or flameproof casserole over medium-high heat. Add the zucchini and cook, stirring occasionally, until beginning to brown, about 3 minutes. Add the onion and garlic and cook, stirring occasionally, until the onions soften, about 2 minutes. Stir in the tomatoes and cook just until they are warm, about 1 minute. Season with the salt and pepper. Transfer to a bowl.

Meanwhile, bring the broth and water to a boil in a medium saucepan over high heat. Reduce the heat to very low to keep the broth mixture warm.

Heat the remaining 2 teaspoons oil in the Dutch oven over medium heat. Add the rice and cook, stirring well, until it turns opaque, about 2 minutes. Stir about ¾ cup of the hot broth mixture into the rice. Cook, stirring almost constantly, until the rice absorbs almost all of the broth, about 3 minutes. Add another ¾ cup of broth and stir until it is almost absorbed. Repeat, keeping the risotto at a steady simmer and adding more broth as it is absorbed, until you use all of the broth and the risotto is barely tender, about 20 minutes total. During the last minute of cooking, stir in the zucchini mixture so it can reheat. The risotto should be loose but not soupy. If you run out of stock and the risotto isn't tender, add more hot water. Stir in the oregano and lemon zest.

Divide evenly among four soup bowls and sprinkle each with 1 tablespoon Parmesan cheese. Serve immediately.

NUTRITIONAL ANALYSIS
(1 serving) 280 calories, 10 g protein, 46 g carbohydrates, 7 g fat, 3 g fiber, 4 mg cholesterol, 384 mg sodium, 585 mg potassium. Food groups: 2 grains, 2 vegetables.

Asparagus and Ricotta Polenta Pizza

This is a pretty dish, with green asparagus and white cheese set off by the golden polenta crust. Serve it as a light supper or even as a brunch dish when company comes over.

Olive oil in a pump sprayer

2¼ cups water

½ teaspoon kosher salt

1 cup coarse yellow cornmeal (polenta)

6 ounces asparagus spears, woody ends trimmed

⅓ cup low-fat ricotta

½ cup (2 ounces) shredded reduced-fat mozzarella

1 tablespoon chopped fresh basil or oregano, for serving

Crushed hot red pepper flakes, for serving

Preheat the oven to 425°F. Spray a 9-inch springform pan with oil.

To make the polenta: Bring the water and salt to a boil over high heat in a medium saucepan. Whisk in the cornmeal. Reduce the heat to medium-low and cook, whisking often, until the polenta comes to a boil. Using an oiled rubber spatula, spread the polenta evenly in the springform pan.

Bake until the polenta is firm and beginning to brown, about 30 minutes. Remove from the oven. Run a sharp knife around the inside of the pan to loosen the polenta.

To make the pizza: Spread the asparagus on a rimmed baking sheet and spray with oil. Bake until the asparagus is crisp-tender, about 4 minutes.

Dollop heaping teaspoons of the ricotta over the polenta. Top with the asparagus, and sprinkle with the mozzarella. Return to the oven and bake just until the mozzarella melts, about 5 minutes. Remove the sides of the pan. Sprinkle the pie with the basil and hot pepper. Cut into six wedges and serve hot.

NUTRITIONAL ANALYSIS
(1 serving) 108 calories, 5 g protein, 18 g carbohydrates, 2 g fat, 2 g fiber, 6 mg cholesterol, 200 mg sodium, 143 mg potassium. Food groups: 1 whole grain, 1 vegetable, ½ dairy.

Side Dishes

Don't let side dishes be an afterthought in your menus. It is easy to get into a rut with this category, so I have created more interesting versions of old favorites. Look for ways to combine two food groups in a single dish, such as kale and beans or carrots and edamame. Or add nuts to increase the protein in a vegetable dish, as I have done to dress up the Brussels sprouts and summer squash recipes. Above all, don't be afraid of a little butter. One tablespoon in a recipe that serves four to six people isn't much, and the flavor payoff is worth the extra few fat grams. More important, the fat helps your body absorb the vegetables' nutrients.

Black Beans and Brown Rice

Don't serve plain white rice when you can offer this nutritious version with Latino flavors. Even if you leave out the black beans and cilantro, this is still a great way to dress up brown rice.

MAKES 6 SERVINGS

2 teaspoons olive oil

1 small yellow onion, finely chopped

1 clove garlic, minced

½ cup long-grain brown rice

1½ cups water

½ teaspoon kosher salt

1 (15-ounce) can reduced-sodium black beans, drained and rinsed

2 tablespoons finely chopped fresh cilantro

Heat the oil in a small saucepan over medium heat. Add the onion and garlic and cook, stirring occasionally, until tender, about 5 minutes. Add the rice and stir well.

Stir in the water and salt and bring to a boil. Reduce the heat to low and cover tightly. Simmer until the rice is tender and almost all the liquid has been absorbed, about 40 minutes. Add the beans, but do not stir them into the rice. Cover the saucepan again and cook until the liquid is absorbed and the beans are hot, about 5 minutes. Remove from the heat and let stand for 5 minutes.

Stir in the cilantro with a fork, fluffing the rice as you do so. Transfer to a serving bowl and serve hot.

NUTRITIONAL ANALYSIS
(1 serving) 139 calories, 4 g protein, 27 g carbohydrates, 2 g fat, 4 g fiber, 0 mg cholesterol, 299 mg sodium, 339 mg potassium. Food groups: 1 whole grain, 1 beans.

Quick "Baked" Beans

Baked beans is a favorite side dish, but it can take a long time to cook. Here is my quick stovetop version, with apples and red bell pepper to increase the fruit and vegetable servings.

MAKES 6 SERVINGS

1 strip reduced-sodium bacon, coarsely chopped

1 teaspoon canola oil

1 small yellow onion, chopped

1 small red bell pepper, cored and cut into ½-inch dice

1 Granny Smith apple, cored and cut into ½-inch dice

1 (15-ounce) can no-salt-added cannellini beans, drained and rinsed

2 tablespoons no-salt-added tomato ketchup

1 tablespoon amber agave nectar, maple syrup, or honey

1 tablespoon cider vinegar

Cook the bacon and oil together in a medium saucepan over medium heat, stirring occasionally, until crisp and browned, about 6 minutes. Add the onion, bell pepper, and apple and cook, stirring occasionally, until the onion softens, about 5 minutes.

Stir in the beans, ketchup, agave, and vinegar. Cook, stirring occasionally, until the sauce has thickened slightly, about 10 minutes. Serve hot.

NUTRITIONAL ANALYSIS

(1 serving) 183 calories, 8 g protein, 32 g carbohydrates, 3 g fat, 6 g fiber, 5 mg cholesterol, 80 mg sodium, 546 mg potassium. Food groups: 1 beans, 1 fruit, 1 vegetable.

Baby Bok Choy and Shiitake Mushrooms

This is an outstanding side dish for simply prepared meat, poultry, or seafood. Baby bok choy and shiitake mushrooms were once available only at Asian markets, but now most supermarkets carry them. MAKES 4 SERVINGS

2 teaspoons canola or corn oil

8 shiitake mushrooms, stems discarded, cut in half vertically

1 scallion, white and green parts, finely chopped

1 tablespoon unpeeled finely shredded fresh ginger

2 cloves garlic, minced

6 baby bok choy (6 ounces), well rinsed

½ cup Homemade Chicken Broth (page 38) or canned low-sodium chicken broth

¼ cup plus 1 tablespoon water

2 teaspoons reduced-sodium soy sauce

⅛ teaspoon crushed hot red pepper flakes

1 teaspoon cornstarch

Heat the oil in a large nonstick skillet over medium-high heat. Add the mushrooms and cook, stirring occasionally, until lightly browned, about 6 minutes.

Add the scallion, ginger, and garlic and stir until fragrant, about 30 seconds. Arrange the bok choy in the skillet. Add the broth, the ¼ cup water, soy sauce, and hot pepper and bring to a simmer. Reduce the heat to low and cover. Simmer until the bok choy is just tender when pierced with the tip of a small, sharp knife, 7 to 10 minutes.

Using a slotted spoon, transfer the vegetable mixture to a serving bowl. Pour the remaining 1 tablespoon water into a ramekin or custard cup, sprinkle in the cornstarch, and stir until dissolved. Whisk into the skillet and bring to a simmer to thicken the sauce. Pour any juices from the serving bowl into the skillet and whisk. Pour the sauce over the vegetables and serve hot.

NUTRITIONAL ANALYSIS

(1 serving) 53 calories, 3 g protein, 6 g carbohydrates, 3 g fat, 2 g fiber, 0 mg cholesterol, 246 mg sodium, 322 mg potassium. Food groups: 1½ vegetables.

Broccoli Ziti

You can enjoy pasta on the **DASH** diet, and it is even better augmented by plenty of vegetables. This mixture is versatile and goes well with the Italian-style red sauces that everyone loves.   MAKES 6 SERVINGS

1 tablespoon olive oil

1 clove garlic, minced

1 broccoli head (about 14 ounces)

1½ cups ziti or other tubular pasta

Pinch of kosher salt

Pinch of freshly ground black pepper

Bring a large pot of water to a boil over high heat.

Heat the oil and garlic together in a small skillet over medium heat, stirring often, until the garlic is softened and fragrant, but not browned, about 2 minutes. Remove from the heat and set aside.

Trim the broccoli, cutting the florets from the stalks. Peel the stalks with a vegetable peeler (don't worry about getting every bit of the peel off) and cut crosswise into ¼-inch-thick slices. Cut the florets into bite-sized pieces.

Add the broccoli to the boiling water and cook until crisp-tender, about 5 minutes. Using a wire sieve or a skimmer, transfer the broccoli to a bowl. Leave the water boiling.

Add the ziti and cook according to the package directions until al dente. During the last minute, return the broccoli to the water. Drain the ziti and broccoli and transfer to a serving bowl. Stir in the garlic-oil mixture, salt, and pepper. Serve hot.

NUTRITIONAL ANALYSIS
(1 serving) 122 calories, 5 g protein, 20 g carbohydrates, 3 g fat, 2 g fiber, 0 mg cholesterol, 56 mg sodium, 259 mg potassium. Food groups: 1 grain, 1 vegetable.

Variation

Green Beans and Fusilli: Substitute 10 ounces green beans, trimmed and cut into 1-inch pieces, for the broccoli; and substitute short fusilli for the ziti.

NUTRITIONAL ANALYSIS
(1 serving) 120 calories, 4 g protein, 21 g carbohydrates, 3 g fat, 2 g fiber, 0 mg cholesterol, 38 mg sodium, 189 mg potassium. Food groups: 1 grain, 1 vegetable.

Broccoli Rabe with Pine Nuts

The brawny flavor of broccoli rabe (also called rapini) meets its match with garlic and vinegar and then gets a crunchy, sweet note from pine nuts. As with many other greens, the amount of time required to cook the broccoli rabe is up to you. Fifteen minutes is about average; you can cook for as little as 5 minutes or as long as 30 minutes.

MAKES 4 SERVINGS

1 bunch broccoli rabe, coarsely chopped into ¾-inch-wide pieces

¼ cup pine nuts

2 teaspoons olive oil

2 cloves garlic, minced

2 teaspoons red wine vinegar

¼ teaspoon kosher salt

Rinse the broccoli rabe well in a large bowl of cold water, then lift the pieces out of the water, leaving any grit behind in the bowl, and transfer to another bowl; do not drain.

Heat a nonstick medium skillet over medium heat. Add the pine nuts and cook, stirring occasionally, until toasted, about 2 minutes. Transfer the nuts to a small plate.

Cook the oil and garlic in the skillet over medium heat, stirring often, until the garlic softens, about 1 minute. In batches, add the broccoli rabe and any clinging water to the skillet. Cover and cook, stirring occasionally, until tender, about 15 minutes. Stir in the vinegar. Season with the salt, and stir in the pine nuts. Transfer to a serving bowl and serve hot.

NUTRITIONAL ANALYSIS
(1 serving) 105 calories, 5 g protein, 5 g carbohydrates, 9 g fat, 3 g fiber, 0 mg cholesterol, 161 mg sodium, 281 mg potassium. Food groups: 1 vegetable, 1 fat.

Roasted Brussels Sprouts with Toasted Almonds

There used to be one way to cook Brussels sprouts: boiling. Now, most cooks have discovered how well roasting complements them. Try these with sautéed pork chops.

MAKES 4 SERVINGS

Olive oil in a pump sprayer

10 ounces Brussels sprouts, trimmed and halved

¼ cup sliced almonds, toasted (see "Toasting Nuts," page 60)

1 tablespoon sherry vinegar

⅛ teaspoon freshly ground black pepper

Preheat the oven to 400°F. Spray a large baking sheet with oil.

Spread the Brussels sprouts on the baking sheet and spray them with oil. Bake, stirring occasionally, until barely tender with browned edges, 30 to 40 minutes.

Transfer to a serving dish. Sprinkle with the almonds, vinegar, and pepper and toss. Serve hot.

NUTRITIONAL ANALYSIS
(1 serving) 70 calories, 4 g protein, 8 g carbohydrates, 4 g fat, 4 g fiber, 0 mg cholesterol, 18 mg sodium, 324 mg potassium. Food groups: 1½ vegetables, ¼ nuts.

Baby Carrots and Edamame with Ginger-Lime Butter

Why have plain baby carrots when you can jazz them up with edamame and a quick sauce? I often cook with a bit of butter, which can make the difference in a dish.

MAKES 4 SERVINGS

8 ounces baby-cut carrots

1 cup thawed frozen edamame

2 teaspoons unsalted butter

2 teaspoons peeled and minced fresh ginger

Freshly grated zest of ½ lime

1 tablespoon fresh lime juice

Pinch of kosher salt

Pinch of freshly ground black pepper

Bring a medium saucepan of water to a boil over high heat. Add the carrots and cook until almost tender, about 6 minutes. Add the edamame and cook until heated through, about 2 minutes more. Drain in a colander.

Cook the butter and ginger together in the saucepan over medium heat, stirring often, until the ginger softens, about 2 minutes. Add the vegetables, lime zest and juice, salt, and pepper and mix well. Transfer to a serving bowl and serve hot.

NUTRITIONAL ANALYSIS
(1 serving) 72 calories, 3 g protein, 8 g carbohydrates, 3 g fat, 3 g fiber, 5 mg cholesterol, 96 mg sodium, 289 mg potassium. Food groups: ½ beans, ½ vegetable.

Roasted Cauliflower with Sage

Like its cousin Brussels sprouts, cauliflower is even better when roasted instead of boiled. Once you have experienced golden-brown, crisp-tender, and fresh-tasting roasted cauliflower, you may never go back to cooking it the old way.   MAKES 6 SERVINGS

1 tablespoon olive oil, preferably extra-virgin, plus more in a pump sprayer

1 cauliflower (about 1¼ pounds)

1 clove garlic, minced

2 tablespoons finely chopped fresh sage

Preheat the oven to 400°F. Spray a large rimmed baking sheet with oil.

Trim the cauliflower and break into bite-sized florets. Spread on the baking sheet and spray with oil. Bake, stirring occasionally, until crisp-tender and lightly browned around the edges, about 30 minutes.

Meanwhile, bring the 1 tablespoon oil and garlic to a simmer in a small saucepan. Remove from the heat and set aside.

Remove the cauliflower from the oven. Add the garlic-oil and sage and mix well. Transfer to a serving dish and serve hot.

NUTRITIONAL ANALYSIS
(1 serving) 35 calories, 2 g protein, 5 g carbohydrates, 1 g fat, 2 g fiber, 0 mg cholesterol, 28 mg sodium, 286 mg potassium. Food groups: 1 vegetable.

Collard Greens with Bacon

Collard greens are usually cooked with pork, as the fat helps improve the absorption of the greens' nutrients. A little reduced-sodium bacon does the trick here. Most supermarkets now carry 1-pound bags of chopped collard greens. Just because they are bagged does not mean they do not have to be cleaned, so rinse well before using.   MAKES 4 SERVINGS

2 slices reduced-sodium bacon, coarsely chopped

1 teaspoon vegetable oil

1 medium yellow onion, chopped

2 cloves garlic, minced

1 (1-pound) bag chopped collard greens, rinsed, but not dried

½ cup water

½ teaspoon crushed hot red pepper

2 teaspoons cider vinegar

Cook the bacon and oil in a large saucepan over medium heat, stirring often, until the bacon is crisp and browned, about 6 minutes. Add the onion and cook, stirring occasionally, until golden, about 5 minutes. Stir in the garlic and cook until fragrant, about 30 seconds.

In batches, stir in the collard greens with any clinging water and cover, letting the first batch wilt before adding another. Add the water and hot pepper. Reduce the heat to medium-low and cover. Cook, stirring occasionally, until the collard greens are very tender, about 30 minutes. Stir in the vinegar.

Transfer the collard greens and any cooking liquid to a serving dish and serve hot.

NUTRITIONAL ANALYSIS
(1 serving) 114 calories, 6 g protein 10 g carbohydrates, 4 g fat, 4 g fiber, 8 mg cholesterol, 116 mg sodium, 136 mg potassium. Food groups: 2 vegetables, 1 fat.

Corn and Tomato Sauté

It is fun to eat corn on the cob, but for a more upscale version, cut the kernels off the ears and sauté them with cherry tomatoes. This vegan dish, high in potassium and fiber, is really best with summer corn and tomatoes, although it is also a good way to improve on frozen corn.

MAKES 4 SERVINGS

Olive oil in a pump sprayer

1½ cups fresh corn kernels (from 3 ears of corn)

1 cup cherry or grape tomatoes, cut in halves crosswise

1 tablespoon finely chopped shallot

½ teaspoon finely chopped fresh thyme, or ¼ teaspoon dried thyme

¼ teaspoon kosher salt

⅛ teaspoon freshly ground black pepper

Spray a large nonstick skillet with oil and heat over medium-high heat. Add the corn and cook, stirring occasionally, until the kernels begin to brown, about 5 minutes.

Stir in the tomatoes, shallot, thyme, salt, and pepper and cook, stirring often, until the tomatoes are heated through, about 3 minutes. Serve hot.

NUTRITIONAL ANALYSIS

(1 serving) 233 calories, 13 g protein, 39 g carbohydrates, 5 g fat, 9 g fiber, 0 mg cholesterol, 180 mg sodium, 1,082 mg potassium. Food groups: 2 grains, ½ vegetable.

Corn and Vegetable Pudding

Most renditions of this dish are laden with cream and cheese, but here the vegetables are allowed to be the star. MAKES 6 SERVINGS

2 teaspoons canola oil, plus more in a pump sprayer

1 medium red bell pepper, cored and cut into ½-inch dice

2 scallions, white and green parts, finely chopped

1 clove garlic, minced

½ jalapeño, seeded and minced

2 cups fresh corn kernels (cut from 3 large ears of corn)

2 teaspoons cornstarch

1 cup low-fat (1%) milk

1 large egg plus 2 large egg whites

½ teaspoon kosher salt

¼ teaspoon freshly ground black pepper

Preheat the oven to 350°F. Spray a 1½-quart or 2-quart round baking dish with canola oil.

Heat the 2 teaspoons oil in a medium nonstick skillet over medium heat. Add the bell pepper, scallions, garlic, and jalapeño and cook, stirring often, until the bell pepper is tender, about 5 minutes. Add the corn kernels and cook, stirring often, until heated through, about 5 minutes. Transfer to a medium bowl and let cool slightly.

Sprinkle the cornstarch over the milk in a medium bowl and whisk to dissolve. Add the egg, egg whites, salt, and pepper and whisk together. Pour over the corn mixture and stir well. Pour into the baking dish.

Bake just until a knife inserted in the center of the pudding comes out clean, about 30 minutes. Let stand for 5 minutes, then serve hot.

NUTRITIONAL ANALYSIS
(1 serving) 98 calories, 5 g protein, 13 g carbohydrates, 3 g fat, 2 g fiber, 33 mg cholesterol, 212 mg sodium, 374 mg potassium. Food groups: 1 whole grain.

Italian Kale and White Beans

The Italian way to prepare kale uses plenty of garlic, and beans are sometimes tossed into the pot, too. For the most authentic flavor, use Tuscan kale (also called *cavolo nero*, or dinosaur kale), with pointed dark green leaves. This vegan dish is full of fiber and potassium.

MAKES 4 SERVINGS

1 tablespoon olive oil

1 medium yellow onion, chopped

3 cloves garlic, minced

1 pound dark kale

¼ teaspoon kosher salt

⅛ teaspoon crushed hot red pepper

1 (15-ounce) can no-salt-added cannellini beans, drained and rinsed

1 tablespoon red wine vinegar

Heat the oil in a large saucepan over medium heat. Add the onion and garlic and cook, stirring often, until the onion is translucent, about 5 minutes.

Meanwhile, pull off and discard the thick stems from the kale. Taking a few pieces at a time, stack the kale and coarsely slice crosswise into ½-inch-thick strips. Transfer to a large bowl of cold water and agitate to loosen any grit. Lift the kale out of the water, leaving behind any dirt. Do not dry the kale.

Add the kale, salt, and hot pepper to the saucepan. Cover and cook, stirring occasionally, until the kale is almost tender, about 10 minutes. Stir in the beans and cook, stirring occasionally, until the kale is tender and the beans are heated through, about 5 minutes. Remove from the heat and stir in the vinegar. Serve hot.

NUTRITIONAL ANALYSIS
(1 serving) 233 calories, 13 g protein, 39 g carbohydrates, 5 g fat, 9 g fiber, 0 mg cholesterol, 180 mg sodium, 1,082 mg potassium. Food groups: 2 vegetables, 1 bean.

Roasted Mushrooms with Thyme and Garlic

The garlicky, herbaceous aroma of these earthy mushrooms promises great flavor, and they do more than deliver. You'll find yourself making them for much more than a side dish, as they can be used as an omelet filling (page 6) or an addition to salad.

MAKES 4 SERVINGS

2 (10-ounce) containers white mushrooms, quartered (small mushrooms can be halved)

2 tablespoons extra-virgin olive oil

1 teaspoon finely chopped fresh thyme

½ teaspoon kosher salt

¼ teaspoon freshly ground black pepper

2 garlic cloves, thinly sliced

Preheat the oven to 400°F.

Mix the mushrooms, oil, thyme, salt, and pepper in a large bowl to coat the mushrooms. Spread on a large rimmed baking sheet. Bake the mushrooms, stirring occasionally, until they are tender and beginning to brown, about 25 minutes. Tuck the garlic slices under the mushrooms (where they will be protected and not burn) and cook until the garlic softens, about 5 minutes more. Serve hot.

NUTRITIONAL ANALYSIS
(1 serving) 94 calories, 5 g protein, 5 g carbohydrates, 7 g fat, 2 g fiber, 0 mg cholesterol, 253 mg sodium, 460 mg potassium. Food groups: 1 vegetable, 1 fat.

Smashed Yukon Golds with Buttermilk and Scallions

Everyone needs a reliable mashed potato recipe, and this one is especially tasty with tangy buttermilk and browned scallions. You can peel the potatoes if you wish, but I prefer them with the skins left on for added color and texture (and nutrition). While the potatoes are cooking, put the measured buttermilk by the stove to lose its chill. Cold buttermilk makes for cold smashed potatoes.   MAKES 6 SERVINGS

2 pounds Yukon Gold potatoes, scrubbed but unpeeled

1 tablespoon unsalted butter

2 scallions, white and green parts, finely chopped

⅓ cup buttermilk, at room temperature

½ teaspoon kosher salt

¼ teaspoon freshly ground black pepper

Put the potatoes in a medium saucepan and add enough cold water to cover by 1 inch. Cover the saucepan and bring to a boil over high heat. Reduce the heat to medium and set the lid ajar. Cook until the potatoes are tender when pierced with the tip of a sharp knife, about 25 minutes. Drain well and return to the saucepan. Do not peel the potatoes.

Melt the butter in a small nonstick saucepan over medium-high heat. Add the scallions and cook, stirring occasionally, until they begin to brown, about 3 minutes. Add to the potatoes.

Using a potato masher or a large slotted spoon, coarsely mash the potatoes, adding the buttermilk. Season with the salt and pepper. Transfer to a serving bowl and serve hot.

NUTRITIONAL ANALYSIS

(1 serving) 136 calories, 3 g protein, 27 g carbohydrates, 2 g fat, 3 g fiber, 5 mg cholesterol, 176 mg sodium, 655 mg potassium. Food groups: 2 starchy vegetables.

Basic Brown Rice

For a versatile, everyday side dish, whole-grain brown rice is a good choice because it is more filling than processed white rice. Brown rice does take longer to cook than white rice, so keep that in mind. Or cook and freeze a large batch of brown rice when you have extra time, and reheat it in the microwave in a covered microwave-safe bowl.

MAKES 4 SERVINGS

1 cup brown rice
1 dried bay leaf
2 cups water

Bring the rice, bay leaf, and 2 cups of water to a boil in a small heavy-bottomed saucepan over high heat. Reduce the heat to medium-low and tightly cover the saucepan. Simmer, without stirring the rice, until it is tender and has absorbed the water, about 40 minutes. If the water evaporates before the rice is tender, add 2 tablespoons hot water to the saucepan (do not stir it in). Remove from the heat and let stand for 5 minutes.

Fluff the rice with a fork. Discard the bay leaf. If any water remains in the saucepan when the rice is tender, drain the rice in a wire sieve. Serve hot.

NUTRITIONAL ANALYSIS
(1 serving: ½ cup) 108 calories, 3 g protein, 22 g carbohydrates, 1 g fat, 2 g fiber, 0 mg cholesterol, 5 mg sodium, 42 mg potassium. Food groups: 1 whole grain.

Indian Rice with Cashews, Raisins, and Spices

Add a little spice to your rice with this Indian-inspired side dish. If you have turmeric, use it to give the rice a beautiful yellow color. And I love using basmati rice in this recipe. It seems "ricier" than regular rice.

MAKES 4 SERVINGS

2 teaspoons canola oil

1 small yellow onion, finely chopped

1 teaspoon peeled and minced fresh ginger

1 small clove garlic, minced

⅔ cup basmati rice

¼ teaspoon ground turmeric (optional)

1 (2-inch) piece cinnamon stick, or ⅛ teaspoon ground cinnamon

⅛ teaspoon ground coriander

⅛ teaspoon freshly ground black pepper

1⅓ cups Homemade Chicken Broth (page 38) or canned low-sodium chicken broth

⅓ cup coarsely chopped unsalted cashews

¼ cup dark raisins

Heat the oil in a medium saucepan over medium heat. Add the onion, ginger, and garlic and sauté, stirring often, until softened, about 3 minutes. Add the rice, turmeric (if using), cinnamon, coriander, and pepper and stir for 30 seconds. Add the broth and bring to a simmer.

Reduce the heat to medium-low and tightly cover the saucepan. Cook until the liquid is absorbed and the rice is tender, about 20 minutes.

Remove the saucepan from the heat. Add the cashews and raisins, but do not stir them in. Cover the saucepan and let stand for 5 minutes. Fluff the rice with a fork, stirring in the cashews and raisins. Transfer to a serving bowl and serve at once.

NUTRITIONAL ANALYSIS
(1 serving) 311 calories, 8 g protein, 41 g carbohydrates, 13 g fat, 2 g fiber, 0 mg cholesterol, 30 mg sodium, 435 mg potassium. Food groups: 2½ grains, 1 nuts.

Quinoa with Broccoli

Quinoa is especially rich in nutrients when compared with other grains. (Actually, it is neither a grain nor a cereal and is related to spinach.) It stands out among plant sources of protein, since it is a complete protein. It has a higher than average fat content, but it is a healthy fat. Nonetheless, calories are calories, so quinoa is often joined by low-calorie ingredients such as the broccoli in this recipe. Leftovers can be dressed the next day with Lemon Vinaigrette (page 73) as part of a salad.　　　　MAKES 6 SERVINGS

1 broccoli crown (8 ounces), cut into small florets, stalk peeled and chopped

¾ cup quinoa

2 teaspoons olive oil

½ cup finely chopped yellow onion

1 clove garlic, chopped

1½ cups water

½ teaspoon kosher salt

Bring a medium saucepan of water to a boil over high heat. Add the chopped broccoli and cook until crisp-tender, about 4 minutes. Drain and set aside. (There is no need to rinse the broccoli.)

Place the quinoa in a fine-meshed wire sieve and rinse under cold running water to remove its naturally occurring invisible bitter coating. Drain well.

Heat the oil in a medium saucepan over medium heat. Add the onion and garlic and sauté, stirring occasionally, until softened, about 3 minutes. Stir in the quinoa, add the water and salt, and bring to a boil over high heat. Reduce the heat to medium-low and cover tightly. Simmer until the quinoa is tender and has absorbed the liquid, about 20 minutes. (Don't worry if a little liquid remains.)

Remove from the heat and add the broccoli. Do not stir. Cover tightly and let stand for 5 minutes to reheat the broccoli. Fluff the quinoa with a fork and serve hot.

NUTRITIONAL ANALYSIS
(1 serving) 110 calories, 4 g protein, 17 g carbohydrates, 3 g fat, 3 g fiber, 0 mg cholesterol, 180 mg sodium, 261 mg potassium. Food groups: 1 starchy vegetable, 1 vegetable.

Creamed Spinach with Mushrooms

You can have "steakhouse night" with this seemingly sinful classic and the Filet Mignon *au Poivre* with Bourbon-Shallot Sauce on page 81. Or serve it topped with roasted or grilled chicken breast or roasted salmon fillet for a truly delicious meal. Don't bother to use fresh spinach here...frozen works beautifully. MAKES 6 SERVINGS

1 tablespoon unsalted butter

8 ounces white mushrooms, sliced

1 clove garlic, minced

2 (10-ounce) packages thawed frozen spinach, squeezed to remove excess liquid

2 tablespoons cornstarch

2 cups low-fat (1%) milk

½ teaspoon kosher salt

¼ teaspoon freshly ground black pepper

Pinch of freshly grated nutmeg

Melt the butter in a large nonstick skillet over medium-high heat. Add the mushrooms and sauté, stirring occasionally, until beginning to brown, about 8 minutes. Stir in the garlic and cook until fragrant, about 1 minute. Add the spinach and cook, stirring often, to evaporate the excess liquid, about 2 minutes.

In a small bowl, sprinkle the cornstarch over the milk and whisk to dissolve. Stir into the spinach mixture and cook, stirring often, until boiling and thickened, about 2 minutes. Season with the salt, pepper, and nutmeg. Serve hot.

NUTRITIONAL ANALYSIS
(1 serving) 98 calories, 7 g protein, 12 g carbohydrates, 3 g fat, 3 g fiber, 9 mg cholesterol, 272 mg sodium, 573 mg potassium. Food groups: 1½ vegetables, ½ dairy.

Sugar Snap Peas and Lemon Butter

In this side dish, the delicate flavors of sugar snap peas, butter, and chives combine so the whole is greater than the sum of its parts. A little butter (or any oil) helps the body absorb the vegetables' nutrients more efficiently.   MAKES 4 SERVINGS

12 ounces sugar snap peas, trimmed

1 tablespoon unsalted butter

Freshly grated zest of ½ lemon

1 tablespoon fresh lemon juice

1 tablespoon finely chopped fresh chives

Pinch of kosher salt

Pinch of freshly ground black pepper

Bring a medium saucepan of water to a boil over high heat. Add the sugar snap peas and cook until crisp-tender, about 3 minutes. Scoop out and reserve 2 tablespoons of the cooking water. Drain the sugar snap peas in a colander.

Return the sugar snap peas to the saucepan and add the reserved water, butter, lemon zest and juice, chives, salt, and pepper. Mix well, allowing the melting butter to mingle with the water. Transfer to a serving bowl and serve hot.

NUTRITIONAL ANALYSIS
(1 serving) 62 calories, 2 g protein, 6 g carbohydrates, 3 g fat, 2 g fiber, 8 mg cholesterol, 53 mg sodium, 174 mg potassium. Food groups: 1 vegetable, ½ fat.

Summer Squash and Walnut Sauté

Two kinds of squash, green and yellow, are complemented by crunchy walnuts in this quick side dish.

MAKES 6 SERVINGS

1 tablespoon olive oil

½ jalapeño, seeded and minced

1 medium zucchini, cut in half lengthwise and then into ¼-inch-thick slices

1 medium yellow summer squash, cut in half lengthwise and then into ¼-inch-thick slices

¼ cup chopped walnuts

1 clove garlic, minced

Pinch of kosher salt

Heat the oil in a large nonstick skillet over medium-high heat. Add the jalapeño and sauté, stirring often, until softened, about 1 minute.

Add the zucchini and yellow squash and cook, stirring occasionally, until browned and tender, 6 to 8 minutes. Stir in the walnuts, garlic, and salt and cook until the garlic is fragrant, about 1 minute. Serve hot.

NUTRITIONAL ANALYSIS

(1 serving) 61 calories, 2 g protein, 2 g carbohydrates, 5 g fat, 1 g fiber, 0 mg cholesterol, 35 mg sodium, 131 mg potassium. Food groups: 1 vegetable, 1 fat.

Squash and Bell Pepper Casserole

Here is an old-fashioned vegetable dish that everyone knows and loves, with extra flavor from green peppers and Italian seasonings. To save washing an extra pan, use an ovenproof skillet that can perform double duty.   MAKES 4 SERVINGS

1 tablespoon plus
1 teaspoon olive oil

2 medium yellow squash,
cut in half lengthwise and
then into ½-inch-thick
slices

1 small yellow onion,
chopped

½ medium green bell
pepper, cored and cut
into ½-inch dice

1 teaspoon Italian
Seasoning (page xiv)

1 clove garlic, minced

¼ cup panko (Japanese-
style bread crumbs),
preferably whole-wheat
panko (see page 140)

Preheat the oven to 350°F.

Heat the 1 tablespoon oil in an ovenproof medium nonstick skillet over medium heat. Add the yellow squash and sauté, stirring often, until it is beginning to soften, about 2 minutes. Add the onion and bell pepper and cook, stirring occasionally, until the onion is tender, about 5 minutes. Stir in the Italian Seasoning.

In a small bowl, stir in the remaining 1 teaspoon oil and the garlic. Add the panko and mix well. Sprinkle evenly over the squash mixture.

Bake until the squash is tender, about 15 minutes. Serve hot from the skillet.

NUTRITIONAL ANALYSIS
(1 serving) 84 calories, 2 g protein, 9 g carbohydrates, 5 g fat, 2 g fiber, 0 mg cholesterol, 15 mg sodium, 281 mg potassium. Food groups: 2 vegetables, 1 fat.

Sweet Potato Steak Fries

Orange sweet potatoes (also called yams) add color and flavor to everyday meals. Roasted at high temperature, they can be ready for serving in a surprisingly short time. (A true sweet potato, also called batata or boniato, has yellow flesh and isn't as sweet as the orange variety.) If you want to add a bit of spice, substitute 1 teaspoon chili powder for the black pepper. Note that sweet potatoes count as vegetable servings, and they have the calories of starchy foods. If you are tracking servings, count it under both categories (that is, 2 starches and 2 vegetables). **MAKES 6 SERVINGS**

Olive oil in a pump sprayer

3 large orange-fleshed sweet potatoes (1½ pounds)

½ teaspoon kosher salt

¼ teaspoon freshly ground black pepper

Preheat the oven to 425°F. Spray a large rimmed baking sheet with oil.

Peel the sweet potatoes and cut each lengthwise into 6 long wedges. Spread in a single layer on the baking sheet. Spray with the oil, toss, and spray again. Bake for 15 minutes. Turn the fries and bake until lightly browned and tender, about 15 minutes more. Season with the salt and pepper, toss well, and serve hot.

NUTRITIONAL ANALYSIS
(1 serving) 148 calories, 3 g protein, 34 g carbohydrates, 0 g fat, 5 g fiber, 0 mg cholesterol, 340 mg sodium, 575 mg potassium. Food group servings: 2 starchy vegetables.

Desserts

Sometimes the best dessert is nothing more than seasonal ripe fruit. When the occasion calls for something more complex, use fruit as the main ingredient to reap its many health benefits. The Make It Your Way Granola on page 8 (much less sugary than commercial versions) can be put to good use in desserts as a cinnamon-spiced topping for a crisp or to layer with juicy fruit and creamy yogurt. These desserts use the minimum amount of such natural sweeteners as honey and agave. (If you want to substitute refined sugars, go ahead, but so many of my students are interested in the natural sweeteners that I have complied with their requests.) So when the mood strikes, treat yourself to a healthful dessert.

Baked Apples Stuffed with Cranberries and Walnuts

This old-fashioned dessert remains a favorite and is never better than when served warm out of the oven on a cool evening. On the other hand, it is also good chilled for breakfast. Be sure to use an apple variety that holds its shape during cooking. The apple farmer at your farmer's market may have some suggestions beyond the two listed here.

MAKES 4 SERVINGS

4 baking apples, such as Braeburn or Rome

½ lemon

⅓ cup dried cranberries

⅓ cup chopped walnuts

6 tablespoons grade B maple syrup (see "Maple Syrup," page 92)

¼ teaspoon ground cinnamon

¼ teaspoon freshly grated nutmeg

4 teaspoons unsalted butter

1 cup boiling water

Preheat the oven to 350°F.

One at a time, cut off the top inch of an apple to make a "lid." Scoop out the core with a melon baller, stopping about ½ inch from the bottom of the apple. Using a vegetable peeler, remove the top half of the apple skin. Rub the exposed flesh all over with the lemon half.

In a medium bowl, mix the cranberries, walnuts, 2 tablespoons of the maple syrup, cinnamon, and nutmeg. Stuff the apples with the mixture. Top each with 1 teaspoon of butter. Replace the apple "lids."

Transfer to a baking dish just large enough to hold the apples. Squeeze the lemon juice from the lemon half over the apples. Pour in the boiling water and cover tightly with aluminum foil. Bake for 20 minutes. Uncover and baste with the liquid in the baking dish. Continue baking until the apples are tender when pierced with the tip of a small, sharp knife, 20 to 30 minutes more, depending on the size of the apples. Remove from the oven and let stand for 5 minutes.

Transfer each apple to a dessert bowl and drizzle each with 1 tablespoon maple syrup. Serve warm.

NUTRITIONAL ANALYSIS

(1 serving) 297 calories, 3 g protein, 54 g carbohydrates, 10 g fat, 5 g fiber, 10 mg cholesterol, 6 mg sodium, 315 mg potassium. Food groups: 1½ fruits, ½ nuts.

Buttermilk *Panna Cotta* with Fresh Berries

Here is a creamy, reduced-fat version of the Italian pudding *panna cotta* made with thick and tangy buttermilk. One word of advice: The buttermilk should be warmed, not heated. Even though *panna cotta* means "cooked cream" in Italian, buttermilk will curdle if overheated. This red, white, and blue dessert is a natural for patriotic holidays such as Independence Day. You will need six 6-ounce ramekins, custard cups, or decorative molds for this recipe.   MAKES 6 SERVINGS

3 teaspoons unflavored gelatin powder

¼ cup plus 2 tablespoons low-fat (1%) milk

2¾ cups buttermilk

½ cup amber agave nectar or honey

½ teaspoon vanilla extract

Canola oil in a pump sprayer

½ cup fresh blueberries

½ cup fresh raspberries

Sprinkle the gelatin over the milk in a small heatproof bowl and let stand until the gelatin absorbs the milk, about 5 minutes. Add enough water to a small skillet to come ½ inch up the sides and bring to a simmer over low heat. Put the bowl with the gelatin mixture in the water and stir constantly with a small heatproof spatula until the gelatin is melted and completely dissolved, about 2 minutes.

Meanwhile, warm the buttermilk in a medium saucepan over medium-low heat, stirring constantly, just until it is warm to the touch. Do not overheat, or it could curdle. Remove from the heat. Add the gelatin mixture and whisk until combined. Whisk in the agave and vanilla. Transfer to a large liquid measuring cup or pitcher.

Oil six 6-ounce ramekins or custard cups. Pour equal amounts of the buttermilk mixture into the ramekins. Cover each with plastic wrap. Refrigerate until chilled and set, at least 4 hours or up to 2 days.

Run a dinner knife around the inside of each ramekin, being sure to reach to the bottom to break the air seal. Working with one *panna cotta* at a time, place a plate over the top of the ramekin. Holding the ramekin and plate together, give them a firm shake to unmold the *panna cotta* onto the plate. If it is stubborn, dip the ramekin (right side up) in a bowl of hot water and hold for 10 seconds, dry the ramekin, invert, and try unmolding again. Sprinkle with the blueberries and raspberries and serve chilled.

NUTRITIONAL ANALYSIS
(1 serving) 148 calories, 5 g protein, 30 g carbohydrates, 1 g fat, 1 g fiber, 5 mg cholesterol, 127 mg sodium, 218 mg potassium. Food groups: 1 dairy, ½ fruit.

Cantaloupe and Mint Ice Pops

You will be happy to have a supply of these ice pops in your freezer for snacking. If you don't have an ice pop mold set (easy to find online and even at supermarkets in the summer), turn the mixture into the granita variation.　　　　MAKES 8 POPS

3 cups peeled, seeded, and cubed ripe cantaloupe

½ cup amber agave nectar

2 tablespoons fresh lemon juice

1 tablespoon finely chopped fresh mint

Have ready eight ice pop molds. Puree 2½ cups of the cantaloupe cubes in a food processor or blender. Transfer to a bowl. Pulse the remaining ½ cup cantaloupe cubes in the food processor or blender (or chop by hand) until finely chopped, and add to the puree. Whisk in the agave, lemon juice, and mint.

Divide the puree among the ice pop molds and cover each mold with its lid. Freeze until the pops are solid, at least 4 hours. (The pops can be stored in the freezer for up to 1 week.)

To serve, rinse a pop mold under lukewarm water and remove the pop from the mold. Serve frozen.

Cantaloupe and Mint Granita: Place a metal baking dish or cake pan and a metal fork in the freezer until very cold, about 15 minutes. Puree all of the cantaloupe. Add the agave and lemon juice and pulse to combine well. Add the mint and pulse just to combine. Pour into the metal dish and freeze until the mixture is icy along the sides of the dish, about 1 hour. Use the cold fork to stir the icy crystals into the center. Freeze again until icy, about 1 hour more, and stir again; the mixture will become more solid. Freeze until the consistency is slushy, about 1 hour more. Freeze until serving, up to 4 hours. Just before serving, use the tines of the fork to scrape the mixture into icy slush. Serve immediately in chilled bowls.

NUTRITIONAL ANALYSIS
(1 serving) 81 calories, 1 g protein, 21 g carbohydrates, 0 g fat, 1 g fiber, 0 mg cholesterol, 10 mg sodium, 165 mg potassium. Food groups: 1 fruit.

Peach and Granola Parfaits

When your sweet tooth aches, you can't make a quicker or more attractive dessert than this parfait. Of course, you can substitute just about any fruit that is ripe and tasty—berries are especially good, and bananas are also great. Greek yogurt is thicker than regular yogurt, and it gives desserts a luscious richness. Even though it appears that this dish is high in carbohydrates, in reality the lactose (milk sugar) in the yogurt has been converted to lactic acid during the ripening process, so it is no longer a carb. MAKES 4 SERVINGS

1 cup plain low-fat Greek yogurt

2 tablespoons amber agave nectar, honey, or grade B maple syrup (see "Maple Syrup," page 92)

¼ teaspoon vanilla extract

8 tablespoons Make It Your Way Granola (page 8)

4 ripe peaches or nectarines, pitted and cut into ½-inch dice

Stir the yogurt, agave, and vanilla in a small bowl.

For each serving, in a large parfait glass or wineglass, layer 1 tablespoon granola, 2 tablespoons yogurt, and one-eighth of the diced peaches, then repeat once more. Serve immediately.

NUTRITIONAL ANALYSIS

(1 serving) 161 calories, 8 g protein, 31 g carbohydrates, 1 g fat, 3 g fiber, 4 mg cholesterol, 25 mg sodium, 457 mg potassium. Food groups: 1 whole grain, ¼ dairy, 1 fruit.

Easy Pear Crisp

Choose juicy pears such as Comice or Anjou for this comforting dessert. Adding the granola at the end of baking ensures a crunchy topping. MAKES 6 SERVINGS

Canola oil in a pump sprayer

5 ripe, juicy pears, such as Comice or Anjou, peeled, cored, and cut into ½-inch pieces

2 tablespoons amber agave nectar or grade B maple syrup (see "Maple Syrup," page 92)

1 tablespoon fresh lemon juice

2 teaspoons cornstarch

½ teaspoon freshly grated nutmeg

1 cup Make It Your Way Granola (page 8)

Preheat the oven to 350°F. Lightly spray an 11 × 8½-inch baking dish with the oil.

Mix the pears, agave, lemon juice, cornstarch, and nutmeg in the baking dish. Bake, stirring after 15 minutes, until the pears are tender and have given off their juices, about 30 minutes. Remove from the oven and sprinkle the granola over the pear mixture. Return to the oven and bake just to heat the granola, about 5 minutes. Remove from the oven and let stand for 5 to 10 minutes at room temperature.

Spoon into dessert bowls and serve warm.

NUTRITIONAL ANALYSIS
(1 serving) 201 calories, 4 g protein, 38 g carbohydrates, 5 g fat, 6 g fiber, 0 mg cholesterol, 7 mg sodium, 292 mg potassium. Food groups: 1 whole grain, 1 fruit.

Roasted Pineapple with Maple Glaze

A delicious fruit dessert like this one doesn't need ice cream or any other high-fat embellishments. Since this has only a few ingredients, be sure each one is top-notch; and use a fully ripened pineapple, deeply flavored grade B maple syrup, and unsalted butter.

MAKES 4 SERVINGS

1 ripe pineapple

Canola oil in a pump sprayer

¼ cup grade B maple syrup (see "Maple Syrup," page 92)

1 tablespoon unsalted butter, melted

Preheat the oven to 425°F.

Using a large, sharp knife, cut the pineapple in quarters lengthwise. Cut each quarter lengthwise to yield 8 wedges. Reserve 4 of the wedges for another use.

Working with 1 pineapple wedge at a time, use a paring knife to cut the flesh from the rind in one piece. Cut the flesh vertically into 5 large chunks, keeping them nestled in the rind.

Arrange the pineapple wedges in a baking dish and spray lightly with oil. Roast until just beginning to brown, about 15 minutes. Whisk together the maple syrup and butter in a small bowl. Brush the mixture over the pineapple and bake until the pineapple is glazed, about 5 minutes more. Transfer to four wide dishes, drizzle with the liquid from the baking dish, and serve hot.

NUTRITIONAL ANALYSIS
(1 serving) 138 calories, 1 g protein, 29 g carbohydrates, 3 g fat, 2 g fiber, 8 mg cholesterol, 4 mg sodium, 171 mg potassium. Food groups: 2 fruits.

Fresh Strawberries with Chocolate Dip

Strawberries and chocolate are old friends. If you are serving this dessert to company, use the big, beautiful strawberries with their stems. Bananas are also wonderful dipped into this chocolate sauce, as are dried apricots.

MAKES 4 SERVINGS

½ cup low-fat (2%) canned evaporated milk

5 ounces bittersweet chocolate (about 60% cacao content), finely chopped

24 strawberries, unhulled

Bring the evaporated milk to a simmer in a small saucepan over medium heat. Remove from the heat and add the chocolate. Let stand until the chocolate softens, about 3 minutes. Whisk until smooth.

Divide the chocolate mixture among four small ramekins. Serve the strawberries with the chocolate mixture for dipping.

NUTRITIONAL ANALYSIS

(1 serving) 229 calories, 5 g protein, 28 g carbohydrates, 14 g fat, 4 g fiber, 3 mg cholesterol, 36 mg sodium, 397 mg potassium. Food groups: 1 fruit, 1 fat, ½ dairy.

Metric Cooking Conversions

Cooking Temperatures	
Fahrenheit	Celsius
300	149
325	163
350	177
375	191
400	204
425	218
450	232
475	246

Volume (used for dry and liquid measures)	
U.S.	Metric
¼ teaspoon	1 milliliter
½ teaspoon	2 milliliters
1 teaspoon	5 milliliters
1 tablespoon	15 milliliters
2 tablespoons	30 milliliters

Fluid Ounces	Milliliter
1	30
2	60
3	90
4	120
5	150
6	180
7	210
8	240

U.S.-Metric Cooking Weight Measurement Conversions

U.S.	Metric, kg
8 ounces (½ pound)	0.23
16 ounces (1 pound)	0.45
1½ pounds	0.68
2 pounds	0.91
2½ pounds	1.13
3 pounds	1.36

U.S. Versus Imperial Measurements

The following information is provided as a point of reference.

In U.S. Measurements	In Imperial Measurements
3 teaspoons = 1 tablespoon	
2 tablespoons = 1 fluid ounce	
8 fluid ounces = 1 cup	10 fluid ounces = 1 cup
2 cups = 1 pint	20 fluid ounces = 1 pint
2 pints = 1 quart	40 fluid ounces = 1 quart
4 quarts = 1 gallon	

NOTE: Typically, U.S. recipes use volume, rather than weight, for most ingredients.

Appendix

General Guidelines for the DASH Diet

The DASH diet is based on research entitled Dietary Approaches to Stop Hypertension, a clinical study that examined the effect on blood pressure of a diet based on a variety of healthy foods. Specifically, the diet is very rich in fruits and vegetables and includes low-fat and nonfat dairy, along with nuts, beans, and seeds, as the key foods; grains (mostly whole grains), lean meats, fish, and poultry, and heart-healthy fats round out the plan. The DASH diet calls for a moderate sodium intake, but the recipes in this cookbook may be adjusted to accommodate your needs if your physician has recommended strict sodium restriction.

The balance of foods in the DASH diet provides you with a diet that is rich in potassium, magnesium, and calcium, which are thought to play an important role in lowering blood pressure. The foods are also rich in important plant nutrients such as vitamins, additional minerals, antioxidants, additional phytonutrients, and fiber.

In addition to providing key nutritional information, our analyses specify which DASH food groups (and how much) make up one serving for each recipe. This can help ensure that you are following the DASH guidelines. Recommended daily servings for the DASH diet meal plan are as follows:

Food Groups	Number of Servings for 1,600- to 3,100-Calorie Diets	Number of Servings for a 2,000-Calorie Diet
Grains and grain products (include at least 3 whole-grain servings each day)	6–12	7–8
Fruits	4–6	4–5

(continued)

Food Groups	Number of Servings for 1,600- to 3,100-Calorie Diets	Number of Servings for a 2,000-Calorie Diet
Vegetables	4–6	4–5
Low-fat or nonfat dairy foods	2–4	2–3
Lean meats, fish, poultry, and eggs	1.5–2.5	2 or fewer
Nuts, seeds, and legumes	3–6 per week	4–5 per week
Fats and sweets	2–4	Limited

Resource Guide

Here are three excellent sites for purchasing a wide range of low-sodium products:

Healthy Heart Market
P.O. Box 74
Big Lake, MN 55309
(763) 262-2020
(888) 685-5988
www.healthyheartmarket.com

Low Salt Market
1014 Adams Circle, C-23
Boulder, CO 80303
(303) 350-7904
www.lowsaltmarket.com

Amazon
www.amazon.com

To learn more about the DASH diet: www.dashdiet.org
The DASH Diet Action Plan and *The DASH Diet Weight Loss Solution* provide everything you need to know to implement the DASH diet for better health and for weight loss.

To link up for frequent updates for DASH, health, and well-being or to learn about new DASH tips and our upcoming events, "Like" the DASH diet Facebook page, or follow me on Twitter.
www.facebook.com/dashdiet
Twitter: @dashdiet

For additional DASH diet recipes, check out several of my favorite sites:

http://www.beefitswhatsfordinner.com

http://www.porkandhealth.org

http://www.fruitsandveggiesmorematters.org/?page_id=5

http://www.ilovecheese.com/recipes.asp

http://www.almondsarein.com/recipes

http://www.michiganbean.org/recipes

http://www.pea-lentil.com/cookbook.htm

http://www.walnuts.org/walnuts/index.cfm/all-recipes

http://www.soyfoods.com/recipes

Acknowledgments

First, I am so grateful to my spectacular agent, Laurie Bernstein, and my fabulous editor, Diana Baroni, for believing in the DASH diet, and taking risks to support my efforts to spread the word about DASH. They jumped at the chance to expand our readers' ability to follow the diet, and pulled out all the stops to make this cookbook happen faster than anyone could have believed. This could not have been possible without the help of their assistants, Marc Haskins and Amanda Englander, respectively, and our wonderful production editor, Tareth Mitch.

And I am so in love with Rick Rodgers as a partner in developing this cookbook and all the recipes! We were on a tight schedule and Rick pursued the development with complete passion and professionalism; he is a true force of nature. My thanks to Toni Allegra for organizing and accepting me into the Greenbrier Food Writers' Symposium, where I met Rick and other food writing stars.

Wonderful support was provided by our San Francisco photography team, under the direction of photographer Sheri Giblin, her assistant, Shay Harrington, food stylist Karen Shinto and her assistant, Jeff Larsen, and prop stylist Christine Wolheim.

And I continue to be grateful to organizations for which I have worked that have provided me with the skills and experience to be able to create and communicate, including Nalco Chemical Company, Dominican University (under Judy Beto, PhD, RD), the Cooking and Hospitality Institute of Chicago, and the University of Illinois at Chicago (under Shiriki Kumanyika, PhD, MPH, RD).

I am fortunate to have been taught at an early age how to cook and prepare healthy meals by my mother. And of course, I so much appreciate the steadfast support of my loving husband, Richard.

—Marla Heller

Toni Allegra, director of the Greenbrier Symposium for Food Writers, introduced Marla and me a few years ago when I was a presenter and Marla was an attendee. Toni has made many such felicitous matches, but I want to give her an especially hearty bowl of gratitude and affection.

As usual, my partner Patrick Fisher, and kitchen assistant and dear friend Diane Kniss, were by my side during the recipe development process, helping with shopping, chopping, and cleaning...and eating! Robin Ansell also helped with recipe development. I am also grateful to my literary agent, Susan Ginsburg, and her assistant, Stacy Testa, who are always in there pitching for me.

It was a pleasure working with our photography team: photographer Sheri Giblin, food stylist Karen Shinto and her assistant, Jeff Larsen, and prop stylist Christine Wolheim.

Grand Central Life & Style lavished extra care on this book, and I appreciate the hard work of our editor Diana Baroni, production editor Tareth Mitch, and copy editor Sona Vogel.

—Rick Rodgers

Index

About the Authors

Marla Heller, MS, RD, is a registered dietitian, and holds a master of science in human nutrition and dietetics from the University of Illinois at Chicago (UIC), where she also completed doctoral course work in public health, with an emphasis in behavior sciences and health promotion. She is experienced in a wide variety of nutrition counseling specialties and has taught thousands of people how to adopt the DASH diet. She has been an adjunct clinical instructor in the Department of Human Nutrition and Dietetics at UIC, teaching courses on food science and nutrition counseling. At the University of Illinois Medical Center, she was a dietitian working in the Cardiac Step-Down Unit, the Cardiac Intensive Care Unit, and the Heart-Lung Transplant Unit. She was a civilian dietitian with the U.S. Navy and most recently worked for the U.S. Department of Health and Human Services, including the Healthy Weight Collaborative.

In addition to writing the *New York Times* bestsellers *The DASH Diet Action Plan* and *The DASH Diet Weight Loss Solution*, Marla contributed the four-week menu plan for *Win the Weight Game* by Sarah, the Duchess of York. She has been a featured nutrition expert for many national print, television, radio, Internet, and social media platforms. She is a spokesperson for the Greater Midwest Affiliate of the American Heart Association and a past president of the Illinois Dietetic Association, from which she received their prestigious Emerging Leader Award.

Marla lives with her husband, Richard, and enjoys cooking, gardening, and finding exciting new restaurants.

Rick Rodgers is the author of over forty cookbooks on a huge variety of subjects and a well-known culinary teacher. His work has appeared in *Bon Appétit*, *Food & Wine*, *Fine Cooking*, and on Epicurious.com, and he has been guest chef on many television and radio shows. His website is www.rickrodgers.com.